ROUTLEDGE LIBRA
HEALTH, DISEASE & SOCIETY

Volume 4

HEALTH CARE

HEALTH CARE

Priorities and Management

GWYN BEVAN,
HAROLD COPEMAN,
JOHN PERRIN and RACHEL ROSSER

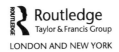

LONDON AND NEW YORK

First published in 1980 by Croom Helm Ltd.

This edition first published in 2022
by Routledge
4 Park Square, Milton Park, Abingdon, Oxon OX14 4RN

and by Routledge
605 Third Avenue, New York, NY 10158

Routledge is an imprint of the Taylor & Francis Group, an informa business

British Library Cataloguing in Publication Data
A catalogue record for this book is available from the British Library

ISBN: 978-0-367-52469-2 (Set)
ISBN: 978-1-032-23498-4 (Volume 4) (hbk)
ISBN: 978-1-032-23535-6 (Volume 4) (pbk)
ISBN: 978-1-003-27812-2 (Volume 4) (ebk)

DOI: 10.4324/9781003278122

Publisher's Note
The publisher has gone to great lengths to ensure the quality of this reprint but points out that some imperfections in the original copies may be apparent.

Disclaimer
The publisher has made every effort to trace copyright holders and would welcome correspondence from those they have been unable to trace.

Health Care Priorities and Management

Gwyn Bevan, Harold Copeman, John Perrin and Rachel Rosser

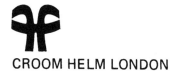

CROOM HELM LONDON

©1980 G. Bevan, H. Copeman, J. Perrin and R. Rosser
Croom Helm Ltd, 2–10 St John's Road, London SW11

ISBN 0 7099 0093 7

Printed in Great Britain by
Redwood Burn Limited
Trowbridge & Esher

CONTENTS

PREFACE

This book follows a research study which three of us, with others, completed in April 1978 at the request of the Royal Commission on the National Health Service.[1] The book has been written before (but will appear after) the publication of the report of the Royal Commission (July 1979–Cmnd 7615) and we have of course been unaware of their views on matters discussed in our text; and the book covers a wider field than our work for them.

The fieldwork for the Royal Commission by the Warwick Team included interviews with staff of Health Departments, three English Regional Health Authorities (RHAs), a single district and a multi-district Area Health Authority (AHA) in each RHA, at least one district of the multi-district AHAs, a Health Board and Health District in Scotland and an AHA and Health District in Wales. The English sample was picked to give a mix of authorities – those gaining or losing under current policies of resource allocation; those with urban or rural areas; and those with teaching or purely service responsibilities. The staff interviewed were mainly concerned with planning, resource allocation, information systems, and budget-holding and financial control. The team also interviewed the chairmen of medical advisory committees and had discussions with authority members and groups of clinicians.

This book explores how the NHS can learn to cope with stresses and problems affecting many countries. Each of the authors, with our different perspectives and experience, knows how difficult it is to establish priorities in the use of public money, and to manage a limited programme when, as in health care, there is always demand for more.

Rachel Rosser, a consultant and senior lecturer in psychiatry at Charing Cross Hospital Medical School, has been working for over ten years on the problems of evaluating the output of health care. Harold Copeman's long experience in the Treasury up to 1976 is directly relevant to appreciating the problems of rationing resources to services in which there is great political interest and economic cost, but for which there is no readily available measure of output. Gwyn Bevan, a lecturer in Operational Research, has been working on the role and limitations of quantitative approaches in the formation of policy through the processes of public planning. John Perrin, a professor of financial control, is concerned with the development of the most appropriate forms of financial procedures and controls so that policy decisions can be taken using relevant financial data, and performance can be monitored and controlled using financial systems. Our joint concern is to suggest ways of enabling realistic and responsible decisions to be taken for achieving the effective use of resources for health care, and to suggest some ways in which the NHS could evolve in a world in which resources are going to fall short of the demands made upon them.

Bevan, Copeman and Perrin were concerned with the research study for the Royal Commission, and are primarily responsible for the text in this book. Dr Rosser has acted as critic and guide and has helped the laymen to see something of the day-to-day and individual problems of doctors working in the NHS.

We are grateful to the Royal Commission for having agreed that (with suitable discretion) we could use our research material for other work which would be published. We are greatly indebted to all those in the NHS who gave their time during the winter of 1977–8, to many friends and colleagues for ideas and advice, and to officials from Government departments who have helped us to bring facts and figures up to date. Crown Copyright material is reproduced with the permission of the Controller of Her Majesty's Stationery Office.

We record our deep gratitude to the secretarial staff of the Centre for Industrial Economic and Business Research, University of Warwick, especially Mrs Norma Bainbridge and Mrs Jane Jordan.

Notes

1. *Management of Financial Resources in the National Health Service,* Royal Commission on the National Health Service, Research Paper No. 2 (Her Majesty's Stationery Office (HMSO), London, 1978).

Abbreviations

We use '£m' for millions of pounds, '£bn' for thousands of millions of pounds. For the UK financial year (e.g. 1978–79, 1 April 1978–31 March 1979) the expression '1978–9' has mainly been used, and (in some quotations) '1978/79'. (In tables of reports, '1978–79' may refer to the session of Parliament.) Abbreviations of names of organisations etc. are explained when first used in the text.

1 INTRODUCTION

Public Expenditure on Health Care – An International Problem

A report in 1977 on *Public Expenditure on Health*[1] in the developed countries of the OECD stated: 'The problems of better controlling and increasing the efficiency and effectiveness of health expenditures are immediate and urgent.' These expenditures by member states in the mid-1970s accounted for 4½ per cent of gross domestic product (GDP) at market prices: they had increased from just over 2½ per cent in the early 1960s, about twelve years before. In the 1970s there had been a particularly explosive increase in several countries which alarmed the governments concerned.

Figures 1.1, 1.2, 1.3 and 1.4 illustrate the growth in expenditure in the UK. Figure 1.1 gives expenditure on the NHS from its first full year (1949) to 1978 at constant prices. This shows nearly unbroken growth in expenditure for the last quarter of a century. Another way of expressing the resource use of the NHS is to put it as a percentage of the national production of resources (GDP). Figure 1.2 gives this ratio and shows the sharp jump in the proportion of the nation's resources expended on the NHS which occurred in the early 1970s. As a consequence of cuts in the growth of public expenditure, the percentage of GDP going into the NHS fell slightly after the peak of 1975. But Figure 1.3 shows that if we consider actual and planned expenditure we can see that the NHS fared better than public expenditure as a whole in the Government's planned restraint.

Figure 1.4 draws all these comparisons together. Expenditure is shown at prices current at the time. As in Figure 1.1 we have used a logarithmic scale so that the steepness of the lines represent their rates of growth at the time. The steepness of the growth in NHS expenditure is striking (line D, from £428m to £7790m – see Table 1 of Appendix). The increase from something over 3 per cent of GDP to around 5 per cent is shown by the movement of line D through the broken lines. For comparison, line C shows general government expenditure on 'goods and services' (including all labour), of which NHS expenditure is an important part. This has varied between 20 per cent and 27 per cent of GDP, without the clear upward trend of the NHS.

However, general government expenditure including benefits and other transfers (line B) rose rather sharply for several years to 1975,

Figure 1.1: NHS Expenditure at 1975 Prices

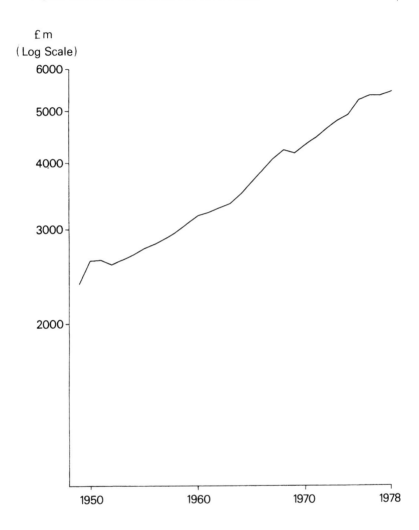

Source: See Table 1 of Appendix.

Figure 1.2: NHS Expenditure as Percentage of GDP (at Market Prices)

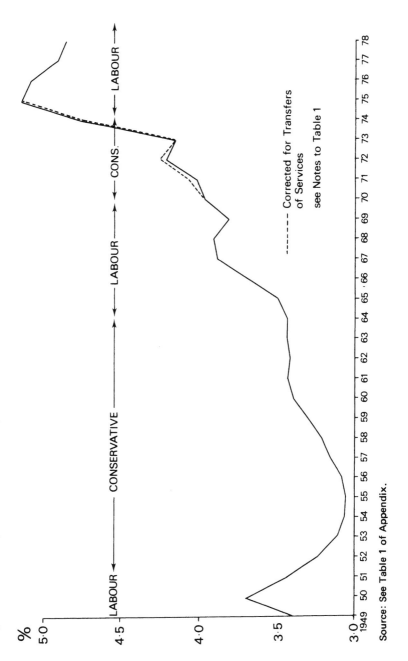

Source: See Table 1 of Appendix.

Figure 1.3: Development in Share of GDP — Health and Total Public Expenditure Based on 1972–3 = 100, and January 1979 Programmes

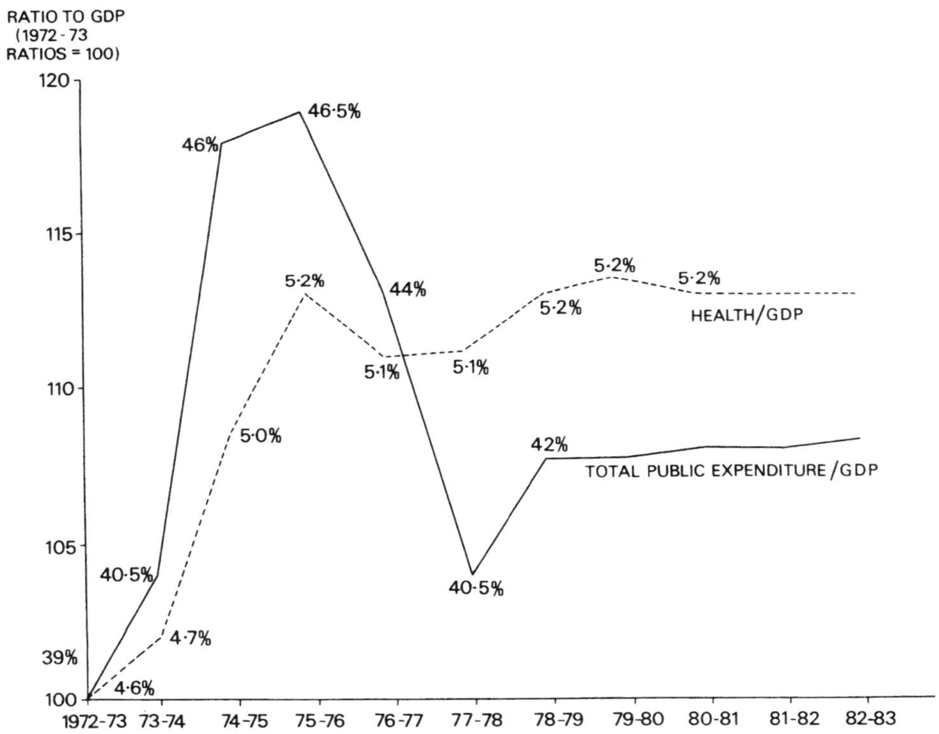

RATIO TO GDP
(1972-73
RATIOS = 100)

HEALTH/GDP

TOTAL PUBLIC EXPENDITURE/GDP

46·5%
46%
44%
40·5%
40·5%
42%

5·2% 5·2%
5·2%
5·2%
5·1%
5·1%
5·2%
5·0%
4·7%
4·6%

120
115
110
105
100
39%

1972-73 73-74 74-75 75-76 76-77 77-78 78-79 79-80 80-81 81-82 82-83

Figure 1.4: NHS Expenditure in Relation to GDP at (GDP Market Prices)

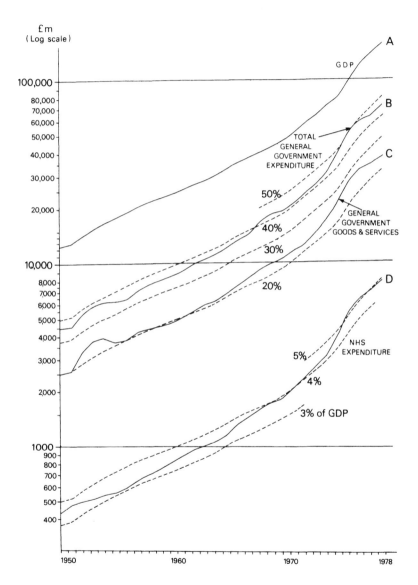

Source: See Table 1 of Appendix.

reaching 50 per cent of GDP, and had to be cut back because of financial crises (see Appendix, Table 2).

The OECD Report reviewed the shift in attitude from the 1960s when a Swedish politician made the often quoted commitment: 'Health care shall cost what it has to cost. We will pay. . . ' By the late 1960s the mood had changed, even in Sweden with its tradition of high public expenditure and taxation. By 1977 governments in the member states of the OECD were tending to decide that increases in expenditure on health care could not be sustained − although this concern was often about unit costs rather than volume. In Belgium a Royal Commissioner was appointed to report on ways to curtail costs. In Canada one of the measures introduced to contain the open-ended nature of expenditure was to link the Federal Government's cost-sharing arrangements to the future GDP growth rate. In the United States President Carter's first policy initiative in health care was to ask Congress to curb the rate of hospital price increases. In Germany a law was introduced to constrain costs of treating sickness.[2]

The OECD Report saw no simple solution to these problems. Experience with charging for treatment and developments of private medicine appear to have little impact in relieving expenditure by the state. The alternative of attempting to achieve a significant reduction in illness by preventing its occurrence seems now to depend on individual rather than state actions.[3]

The report identifies a prevalent fear throughout the governments of the member countries that the 'demand for health services is insatiable on the basis of any pricing system that is socially and ethically acceptable'. It believed that countries will have to set an economic limit on expenditure on health care that will be inadequate to meet demand. The UK has had to meet these pressures already. The Labour Government's policy as explained in the Public Expenditure White Paper of January 1979[4] allowed current expenditure on hospital and community services to grow at an annual average rate of 1.9 per cent up to 1982−3. The Government recognised that for these services 'current expenditure needs to grow at about 1 per cent a year merely to allow for demographic change to make some provision for the spread of improved medical techniques without detriment to standards in other parts of the services'[5]; and as a consequence of this financial restraint 'important unmet needs will remain'.[6]

At the time of going to press, shortly after the new Conservative Government has come into office, there is no reason to expect greatly different policies on health expenditure.

The Need for Health Care Services and Rationing Their Supply

In this book we are concerned with two problems in managing NHS resources. First, there is the difficult matter of deciding what can and cannot be afforded. Proposed developments, even when whittled down to a short list, tend to cost more than the resources likely to be available. Managers of programmes see existing expenditures as having merit, and little scope for savings. On the other hand, people are reluctant to see an explicit price put on health or on saving life. Yet in one way or another we are bound to do this in rejecting new proposals or cutting back on existing expenditures — or indeed in managing any existing programme so as to achieve the best effects for health and life. The second set of problems is concerned with how to plan, to allocate resources and to budget within what can be afforded.

There are various temptations. One may shirk the difficult task of setting priorities, and draw up plans as if there were no resource constraints. One may set next year's budget at the same level as last year's, without looking to see whether resources can be switched. And one may allocate growth money to fund new developments which are decided in a piecemeal manner, without examining the opportunities forgone by these disjointed proposals.

We consider these problems in this book against a complicated and controversial background, even on so basic a question as the effect of medical care on health and life. The Health Departments made the following assessment in 1976:

> . . . the enormous advances in public health during the last century have led to a doubling of the population despite a halving of the birthrate. During the second half of this period, while the expectation of life at early ages has continued to lengthen, the improvement at later stages has been much less — especially for men.
> The chief lesson . . . is the complexity of the reasons for improvements in health. Some diseases have declined for reasons which are still quite obscure. But only to a limited extent and in comparatively recent times can these improvements be clearly attributed to strictly medical activities, such as immunisation or the use of antibiotics. Over the longer term they owe much more to better nutrition, better housing, sanitary engineering, higher standards of personal hygiene and to other wider social and economic changes.[7]

Thomas McKeown has reviewed in detail the impact of medicine on mortality rates compared with environmental and behavioural factors, and concludes that 'medical intervention has made, and can be expected to make a relatively small contribution to prevention of sickness and death'.[8]

An enormous issue remains unresolved. This is the impact of medicine on the relief of sickness, as distinct from prevention of death. McKeown argues, for instance, 'a successful operation which restores the patient to health is not typical of the work of acute hospitals, much of which is palliative or unproved'.[9] He does not suggest that the work of the acute hospital should be dispensed with, but that there must be critical appraisal of the effectiveness and efficiency of medical procedures already in use or to be brought into use. This task is difficult but feasible. It is not possible so far to assess the impact of health care on sickness in the community (morbidity), if only because there is no satisfactory measure of morbidity (see Chapter 8 for a further discussion of this problem).

One set of problems of measuring the effectiveness and efficiency of medical treatment follows from the methodological and ethical difficulties of conducting experiments with the large samples required. A second complication arises from whether there are pressures from society in favour of or against such experiments — after all, it is on the public at large that Randomised Controlled Trials are conducted. Dr David Owen, when Minister of State for Health, attempted to describe the relationship between doctors and society. He suggested that 'Society gives status and privileges to the doctor because people believe in the doctor's ability to heal.'[10] He identified an ambivalent relationship between doctors and society: when we are well we are keen to demystify the doctor's skills, but when we are ill we yearn for belief in the doctor's capacity to heal. Whilst there have been significant advances in medicine in terms of its capacity to save life, improve the quality of life by the relief of suffering and increase the mobility of those with physical disabilities, massive problems remain beyond the scope of medical science:

It is a salutary fact that the vast bulk of modern sickness does not respond to the doctor's skills. The majority of a doctor's time is spent in helping patients to accommodate themselves to the facts of their illness. The largest element in all illness in modern society is the ageing process itself — a largely irreversible process. Health services and the doctors are cast in the role of providers of good health, yet at best, for the bulk of illness all they can do is relieve symptoms. The dramatic cure is the exception rather than the rule.[11]

Until the 1970s we could afford the luxury of belief in the power of the advance of medicine. Now it seems that people in this and perhaps other countries are no longer prepared to continue to finance this advance at the rate of recent years. We must therefore choose the kind of medicine that people are prepared to afford (in the UK mainly through the taxes that they pay). This means, if only there is the courage to do so, a radical but slow and thorough appraisal of the health services now provided, seeking to find ways of using the staff and buildings in the ways that are going to be most effective in the years ahead.

A critical appraisal of current services must impinge upon, and therefore constrain in some way, the doctor-patient relationship in the NHS. This relationship, though resting on a public contract, is private, but rests on social policies and assumptions.

Particularly in our disrupted society[12] there is a compelling need for the idealism of doctors and nurses who provide care, not because, as each service is provided to each patient, an extra item appears on a bill to be eventually settled by the recipient, but solely because the person is in pain and distress and is in need of care. The function of publicly-financed health services is to promise us that when we are ill we will receive care, not according to our ability to pay but according to our need.

The problem that we have to face is that we are not prepared to finance the idealism of doing all that modern medicine could provide for the sick. Resource constraints bite implicitly. Responsibility for these constraints is unclear. Enormous frustration is generated in the NHS by no one knowing at what level these constraints are set. Clarification of responsibility might relieve much of the current frustration, but it requires the courage to make explicit the kind of resource constraints that each level has decided to impose. Until this issue is clearly faced, the line of accountability that runs from the Secretary of State to the doctor will remain long and diffuse. The planning system introduced in England does have the potential of clarifying responsibility, provided that each level does set priorities within available resources and makes explicit what is being forgone.

It is extremely difficult to resolve how rationing ought to work in practice. There are some extreme ideas. Ivan Illich, for example, advocates getting rid of advanced medicine and relying on non-experts.[13] He emphasises the harm that medical treatment can do. There are, however, many effective treatments that do require expertise and do avoid harm – for instance, streptomycin is an effective treatment for tuberculosis but a difficult diagnosis is necessary first: and its side effects are such that its unnecessary prescription should be avoided.[14] We would follow Illich in arguing for more personal responsibility for our health, without agreeing with his polemical attack on the medical profession.

One line of thought which appears to be attractive is to attempt to separate the humane comfort of the suffering from highly expensive medicine practised in an acute hospital. One might, for instance, demand that the latter should prove its value in terms of effectiveness, and leave the former largely unexamined. Unfortunately this is just as illusory as equating effectiveness with simplicity, because it ignores the importance and expense of *diagnosis.* One of the specialties with a recent explosive increase is in the diagnostic services of pathology (see Chapter 2), and currently there is controversy about the highly expensive CAT-scanner being introduced into a number of hospitals, which has the potential of possibly leading to easier diagnosis, and quicker and more effective treatment, and may indeed lead to savings in revenue outgoings. Diagnosis and treatment, furthermore, may well overlap, and the hospital provides a natural extension of the service given by the family practitioner.

Critical appraisal of resource use is likely to bear most heavily on hospital services despite the difficulty of disentangling general practice from the supporting services of the acute hospital. General practice is vital as an immediately accessible service to all in distress without trammels of any kind. Expenditure on hospital services has grown most rapidly. There have been dramatic improvements in making more efficient use of beds, in terms of cases treated, as expenditure has increased, and the increase in staffing may be justified in those terms. We have yet to learn how to evaluate health care, not in terms of cases but in terms of the improvement in health and the cost of securing that improvement. In the end treatment is going to be refused explicitly, not because it does not do any good, but because resources are limited and (given that constraint) there are better ways of using those resources.

In this book we focus on hospital services, though without implying that general practice is unimportant. The scheme of the book is that Chapter 2 gives a historical perspective on rationing for health care; Chapters 3 to 6 describe the organisation and the systems of budgeting, resource allocation, planning, control and monitoring introduced at the 1974 reorganisation (these include a review of different approaches in the different parts of the UK, but focus on the English approach and describe differences from that in the other countries); Chapters 7 to 12, the core of the book, investigate the challenge of rationing, and how the new systems and organisation can measure up to meeting this challenge. We consider that the NHS can expect little more in terms of increases in resources. The chapter on resource allocation describes the problems of rationing on a geographical basis. The chapter on planning describes them in terms of deploying resources and services. The systems of planning and resource allocation are frameworks for making policy decisions. The tasks remain of linking budgeting and financial control to those decisions through the organisational structure. In the two other main chapters we discuss how well the current practices and organisations are designed to perform these tasks and how they might develop to become more effective; and we include a chapter on alternative sources of finance and private medicine. We finish with a chapter of conclusions.

Notes

1. *Public Expenditure on Health, Studies in Resource Allocation,* No. 5 (Organisation for Economic Co-operation and Development (OECD), Paris, 1977).
2. Ibid.
3. See Thomas McKeown, *The Role of Medicine. Dream, Mirage or Nemesis* (Nuffield Provincial Hospitals Trust, London, 1976).
4. *The Government's Expenditure Plans, 1979-80 to 1982-83,* Cmnd 7439 (HMSO, London, 1979), p. 143.
5. Ibid., p. 143.
6. Ibid., p. 139.
7. Health Departments of Great Britain and Northern Ireland, *Prevention and Health: Everybody's Business, A Reassessment of Public and Personal Health* (HMSO, London, 1976).
8. McKeown, *Role of Medicine,* p. 114.
9. Ibid. p. 116.
10. David Owen, *In Sickness and In Health, The Politics of Medicine* (Quartet, London, 1976), p. 88.
11. Ibid., pp. 88-9.
12. Fred Hirsch, *Social Limits to Growth* (Routledge and Kegan Paul, London, 1977).
13. Ivan Illich, *Medical Nemesis* (Calder and Boyars, London, 1975).
14. McKeown, *Role of Medicine,* p. 169.

2 HISTORICAL PERSPECTIVE

For this historical perspective to be of contemporary significance it is helpful to begin by describing the nature of the current rationing problem facing the NHS. Following Tew[1] we can compare the development from 1949 to 1977.

		1949	1977	
There was:				
a. 1 available bed		98	123	
b. 1 in-patient case (discharge/death)		15	9	
c. 1 person on waiting list	for	88	77	persons in the
	every			
d. 1 annual clinic session		46	28	population
e. 1 new out-patient		7	6	
f. 1 new casualty patient		11	5	

B, d, e and f show that in terms of treatment the population was served more intensively by the NHS in 1977 than in 1949, but the proportion of people on the waiting list − c − was virtually the same. Surgical specialties (including gynaecology) account for most of patients waiting for treatment (85 per cent of the total list in 1949 and 95 per cent in 1973). The weighted average time for these specialties initially declined from 117 days in 1949 to 76 days by 1956 and stood at 71 days in 1973. Within this group in 1973 the longest average waiting times were for plastic surgery (268 days), ENT (146 days) and dental surgery/orthodontics (110 days).[2] There has been more efficient and intensive use of resources: these are indicated by reductions in the number of beds − a − and by reductions in length of stay (see later in this chapter). But the reduction in numbers of beds is largely due to closing of beds for tuberculosis and the mentally ill, and the reduction of the average length of stay seems to have flattened out. There may not be much scope for further savings or for significant further reductions in the length of stay. But the core of the problem is that since demand for health care is not self-limiting, but open-ended, increases in supply and/or more efficient use of resources will not in many cases remove excess demand.

The seemingly intractable problem of waiting lists is only the tip of the clinical iceberg of sickness in the community. For a patient to appear on the hospital waiting list he has to both present himself to his general practitioner and be referred to a specialist. In the 1960s some surveys gave some indication of the magnitude of unknown sickness in the community. Last, in 1963,[3] suggested that for every case of diabetes, rheumatism or epilepsy known to the general practitioner, there was another case undiagnosed. Evidence by the British Medical Association (BMA) in 1970[4] brought together a number of such surveys and confirmed Last's findings for these conditions, and suggested that for every known case of psychiatric disorder, bronchitis, urinary infection, high blood pressure and glaucoma, doctors only know of about one case in five. More generally, surveys by Medical Officers of Health, before the 1974 reorganisation, discovered an alarming prevalence of sickness. In Rotherham in 1965, one in six people screened were found to be suffering from one to nine serious illnesses.[5] In Southwark in 1968, in a sample of 1,000, only 67 were found to be completely fit, and 500 were referred to their general practitioner.[6]

Such surveys have been put into perspective by Bradwell *et al.*[7] because they focus on statistical abnormalities rather than illness. It follows, for example, that if (for the sake of argument) abnormality is defined in terms of 5 per cent of the population, then after 15 tests on any patient (assuming independence) it is more likely that not that at least one test will have an abnormal result. This analysis is further weakened because normal values are commonly defined for the population as a whole, not for the patient's particular age and sex group. So 'abnormal' findings may have little to do with the diagnosis of sickness. Indeed, out of 200 patients with 'abnormal' results which could not be explained at the time, a follow-up study five years later found only three to have developed clinical disease which could have been predicted in the earlier survey. Another approach to assessing the degree of sickness in the community is to record self-reported sickness. This approach has been used since the report of the Poor Law Commissioners of 1838.[8] And since 1971 the General Household Survey has conducted analyses of self-reported chronic and acute sickness in a two-week period. In 1976 for example, nearly 25 per cent of the population reported chronic sickness and in the age groups 45–64, 65–74 and over 75 the percentages were 36.6 per cent, 52.1 per cent and 62.6 per cent respectively.[9] The survey published investigated trends in sickness from 1971 to 1976. It reported evidence that suggested the existence of a linear increasing trend in acute sickness among children under 15 of both sexes and females aged 15–44. There was no discernible trend (either decreasing or increasing) among all other age groups of both sexes.[10]

It is extremely difficult to assess what findings about the *stock* of illness in the community mean in terms of the *rate* of treament required to deal with it, if the barriers to ideal treatment were to be removed. One problem is that both 'stock of sickness' and 'available treatments' are dynamic concepts, and change with developments in diagnosis and treatment. These developments mean that even if there were no increase in self-reported sickness there would be an ever-increasing burden. But the General Household Survey has discerned a trend for the rate of self-reported acute sickness to be increasing for certain groups in the community; and, more importantly, the changing population structure will mean a significant increase in demands for health care. Those aged 16 to 64 place comparatively little demand on health services; the heaviest users of services are those aged over 75. In 1977 the DHSS published projections of population growth by age groups from 1976 to 1991. During that 15-year period, live births were forecast to increase by over 30 per cent (children are quite heavy users of health services), those aged 16 to 64 to increase by approximately 5 per cent, those aged over 75 by over 25 per cent, those aged 85 or over by more than 30 per cent.[11]

We delude ourselves if we believe that these problems will be overcome by extra resources. This delusion is dangerous: it is initially comforting, but in the long term is a source of frustration because the promise of amelioration for the deprived parts of the NHS continues to remain a distant prospect. For too long the NHS has striven to achieve an impossible ideal of providing a level of care that could not be financed. Instead of beginning by remedying historic neglect, resources were directed to the already well-endowed.

In 1976 Dr David Owen summarised the inequalities in health care: the faster than average growth in expenditure on teaching hospitals; the geographic inequality in resource allocation; the 'historic and continuing neglect' for services to long-stay patients in hospital, the chronically ill, the mentally handicapped, the elderly, and the young chronic sick.[12] In the same year a departmental working party on resource allocation suggested that in 15 out of 20 teaching hospitals the excess running costs over an equivalent hospital without teaching responsibilities were not explicable in terms of the estimated costs of teaching. The report noted, 'The methods used to distribute financial resources to the NHS have, since its inception, tended to reflect the inertia built into the system by history.'[13] The departmental consultative document on priorities for health and personal social services, also published in 1976,[14] proposed giving priority to services for the elderly, the mentally ill and the mentally handicapped.

In later chapters we amplify these policies, discuss their merit and how the future might be different from the past. If we are to change historic trends it is helpful to understand their origins. This is the purpose of this chapter.

The Cost of an Adequate Service

Reports by Scottish[15] (1977) and English[16] (1976) working parties on methods for moving towards allocating resources on a more equitable basis within each country begin by pointing out that demand will always exceed supply. The Scottish report explains that this contradicts an early belief at the time of the introduction of the NHS. This mistaken belief is put in terms of an initial rapid rise in expenditure which would only require a small future increase 'to satisfy those outstanding needs which were being comparatively ill-served'.[17] This is a diplomatic account of what Ron Brown[18] has described as the egregious error of assuming that NHS expenditure would decline as the existing 'pool of sickness' was gradually mopped up by new services. In this section we explore the nature of early beliefs about NHS expenditure.

The Cost of the Ideal Plan

The Beveridge Report (1942) singled out health care as the outstanding pre-war inadequacy in the provision of social security:

> In one respect only of the first importance, namely limitation of medical service, both in the range of treatment which it is provided as of right and in respect of the classes of persons for whom it is provided, does Britain's achievement fall seriously short of what has been accomplished elsewhere.[19]

Sir William (later Lord) Beveridge advocated revolutionary rather than piecemeal changes in social security. The report stated:

> From the standpoint of Social Security a health service providing full preventive and curative treatment of every kind to every citizen without exceptions, without remuneration limit and without an economic barrier to delay recourse to it is the ideal plan.[20]

The report included 'a very rough estimate' of expenditure in 1945 of £170m, and assumed no change in this figure for the next twenty years because it expected 'some development of the service, and as a consequence of this development a reduction in the number of cases requiring it'.[21] Whilst this appears to be the source of the erroneous assumption about NHS expenditure, it is mistaken and unfair to blame its persistence on one rough estimate in an extended review of plans for social security. The influential *Report on the Future Provision of Medical and Allied Services* (Dawson Report, 1920) analysed the difficulties facing voluntary hospitals at that time, and provided a much sounder guide to future expenditure on the NHS:

> That the hospitals have fallen on evil days is known to all. The reason is two-fold. One is that the prices of all the commodities a hospital has to buy . . . have increased. The other reason is that the investigation and treatment of disease are becoming increasingly complex. So that not only are the old items of expenditure more costly, but there is hardly a year but some new method of diagnosis or treatment makes it necessary to incur fresh expenditure, and capital expenditure in a hospital differs from capital expenditure in business, in that when a hospital grows it grows in spending capacity.[22]

Aneurin Bevan, the minister responsible for the introduction of the NHS, did not believe that expenditure would be self-limiting. Arguments were raised for deferring the introduction of the NHS because existing services would be inadequate to meet demand. These were rejected by Bevan. In speeches to future NHS staff just prior to the Appointed Day (5 July 1948) he said, 'We never will have all we need. Expectation will always exceed capacity'[23] and 'This Service must always be changing, growing and improving, it must always appear inadequate.'[24]

Not only was the assumption of the Beveridge Report of constant or declining future expenditure mistaken: its estimate of initial expenditure turned out to be a gross underestimate. These errors could only help a Minister of Health in gaining Treasury approval for a new National Health Service. It is a well-worn ploy of spending departments to get expenditure proposals through the Treasury by gaining commitment in principle to low initial expenditures which continue to grow but are difficult to stop as they increase – one reason for the introduction of the Public Expenditure Survey in 1961 was to expose this negotiating device by requiring forward projections of expenditure. Undercosting is a second ploy attempted by spending departments in negotiation with the Treasury. The Beveridge Report gave authoritative backing to these well-recognised tactics. Aneurin Bevan 'argued with canny foresight that no worthwhile estimate of the Service's cost could be given until there was practical experience of its working'.[25]

The primary, but not exclusive, concern of the Treasury Supply Division responsible from 1942 to 1948 was to relate the costs of the 1944 White Paper on a National Health Service, and of the 1946 National Health Service Bill, back to the Beveridge Report. (The Treasury were also concerned about statements in the 1944 White Paper which promised to overcome inequalities in access to health services because of the unequal distribution of resources in the UK.[26] We pursue this point later in the chapter.)

The Early Years of the NHS

The mistakes of the Beveridge Report may have eased the introduction of the NHS, but they meant that in its early years its heavy initial expenditure, and continued increase, caused considerable alarm. According to Foot the demand turned out to exceed anything that Bevan had dreamt of.[27] Bevan was subjected to Opposition criticism in the House of Commons. Churchill in the first year of the NHS described the Government's Supplementary Estimate presented to meet expenditure in excess of its initial estimate as 'an event without precedent in time of peace . . . the most wild miscalculations . . . an enormous addition to the burdens of the nation . . . the grossest carelessness'.[28] Supplementary Estimates were again needed for the NHS for 1949–50, and in the debate on the Opposition amendment deploring 'the failure of the Chancellor of the Exchequer to enforce his own instructions to Departments not to overspend so extensively their Estimates',[29] the Chancellor announced that a ceiling on NHS expenditure was to be imposed for 1951–2. As part of this policy, charges for dentures and spectacles were introduced in May 1951 (the decision to do this resulted in the resignation of Aneurin Bevan, Harold Wilson and John Freeman). The newly elected Conservative Government of 1952 reaffirmed the intention to maintain a cash ceiling on health expenditure and introduced further and more extensive charges including a prescription charge. This ceiling was however breached by an award made to general practitioners in 1952, which fulfilled an earlier commitment to maintain the total purchasing power of their income. During that year, a book by Dr Ffrangcon Roberts was published which argued that expenditure on health care was open-ended, and stressed the connection between an ageing population and increased demands for health care.[30] (The Beveridge Report paid considerable attention to the change in structure of the British population which would lead to a greater proportion of elderly in the twenty years following the war, but it only considered their needs in terms of payment of pensions and missed the connection to a growing need for health care.) In reaction to alarm about ever-increasing expenditure on the NHS, the Minister of Health announced the appointment of the Guillebaud Committee in 1953 with the following terms of reference:

> To review the present and prospective cost of the National Health Service; to suggest means, whether by modifications in organisation or otherwise, of ensuring the most effective control and efficient use of Exchequer funds as may be made available, to advise how, in view of the burdens on the Exchequer, a rising charge upon it can be avoided, while providing for the maintenance of an adequate Service; and to make recommendations.[31]

The Findings of the Guillebaud Committee

The committee reported in 1956. Research on the cost of the NHS for the committee by Abel-Smith and Titmuss[32] showed that an over-crude use of the Appropriation Accounts had given a misleading impression of the costs of the Service on four grounds. First, no account was taken of inflation. Second, no distinction was made between capital and current expenditure: fluctuations in the former were treated as changes in consumption. Third, the back pay to doctors of the Danckwerts award of 1952—3 for the earlier years of the service appeared in the accounts for 1952—3 only, giving a misleading impression that the increase over 1951—2 was £40m whereas research showed the underlying increase to be only £8m. Fourth, the net cost, which took account of the charges levied, was, of course, less than the costs as shown by the Appropriation Accounts. The various analyses showed that the NHS was absorbing a decreasing proportion of the nation's resources; that contrary to popular belief, there had not been an increase of vast proportions in either the money cost or the real cost; and that the net diversion of resources from 1949—50 to 1953—4 had been of relatively insignificant proportions.

The research by Abel-Smith and Titmuss examined the components of cost. This analysis is illuminating in terms of the nature of the 'pool of sickness' that had been mopped up by new services. In the first full year of operation (1949—50) the hospital services cost £192m and the executive council services cost £147m. By 1953—4 the former had risen to £263m and the latter had fallen to £123m. The executive council services include general practitioner services by doctors and dentists, and ophthalmic services. Abel-Smith and Titmuss showed that the figures suggested that there had been a backlog of demand for teeth and spectacles and that this demand was declining before charges had been introduced. The increase in hospital expenditure was shown to be due mainly to increased staff and to a lesser extent to increases in supply of medical goods. But these increases could be justified by increased activity in terms of more cases being treated in hospitals, more medical staff being trained, and more research being undertaken.

The committee itself had to make judgements about extravagance, in the demand for health care and inefficiency in its administration. The committee 'found no opportunity for making recommendations which would either produce new sources of income or reduce in a substantial degree the annual cost of the Service',[33] and 'reached the conclusion that the Service's record of performance since the Appointed Day has been one of real achievement. The rising cost of the Service in real terms during the years 1948–54 was kept within narrow bounds; while many of the services provided were substantially expanded and improved during the period. Any charge that there has been widespread extravagance in the National Health Service, whether in respect of the spending of money or the use of manpower, is not borne out by the evidence.'[34] Not only did the committee see no scope for significant savings in expenditure: they also recommended increases in certain instances, in particular in hospital capital expenditure.

Of particular importance was the committee's conclusion that it was quite mistaken to assume that

> the Health Service can and should be self-limiting, in the sense that its own contribution to national health will limit the demands placed upon it to a volume which can be fully met. This at least for the present is an illusion.[35]

One reason was the effects of changes in size and composition of the population. A second concerned changes in the concept of what would constitute an adequate service — even if this could be defined at different times:

> what might have been held to be adequate twenty years ago would no longer be so regarded today, while today's standards will in turn become out of date in the future. The advance of medical knowledge continually places new demands on the Service, and the standards expected by the public also continue to rise.[36]

The Collective Pursuit of the Unattainable

In explaining the opposition of some of the medical profession to the introduction of a national health service Foot offers two explanations. First, at best, this opposition 'derived from a deeply entrenched belief that almost any system of State control would destroy the doctor's clinical freedom'.[37] Secondly, and more fundamentally,

> Many of the spectacular triumphs of British medicine had been won in private practice and in the best voluntary hospitals where leading specialists treated patients who, for the most part could afford to pay . . . How melancholy it would be if these standards were debased, if the vanguard was prevented from making its dashing advance because the whole army must march with it.[38]

Foot then argues that this more fundamental objection was mistaken: in the past the most spectacular triumphs in terms of impact on the health of the nation had been achieved by collective action (e.g. by better drainage, sanitation and water supplies); and that the true principle to be learned from the past and to be applied to the future was to 'carry the power of collective action into the domain of curative medicine'.[39]

Unfortunately the principle does not carry across in any straightforward way. Collective action on the elimination of *infectious* diseases brought *collective* gains. No one could be immune from these diseases, and the elimination of their causes by the improvement in the better living conditions of the poor was in the interests of all. Treatment of noninfectious disease by curative medicine may only benefit the person who receives treatment. In 1911 a national insurance scheme[40] was introduced, for general practice only, which applied to those in work and earning less than a certain income limit — the BMA argued for this limit to ensure private practice for those earning more than the limit.[41] This scheme can be seen as an investment in the working force of the nation where curative medicine could produce benefits beyond those of the person receiving treatment. This argument recurs in the Beveridge Report, which argued for universal coverage for both general practice and hospital treatment as part of the ideal plan from the standpoint of social security, because this would 'increase wealth, by maintaining physical vigour'.[42] The report of the Guillebaud Committee of 1956 pointed out that the NHS could be seen 'as productive' even in the narrow economic sense insofar as it improved the health and efficiency of the working population.[43] And in 1978 *The Way Forward* noted that some Community Health Councils had emphasised the need to maintain services for the economically active population.[44]

The ideal of universal coverage has always proved unattainable because of lack of resources. Before 1948 access was, in the main, rationed by price. The Guillebaud Report can, we suggest, be interpreted as showing that it was likely that health care would always have to be rationed (whether by price or in some other way): demand was not self-limiting, and the changing concept of an adequate service meant continual pressure for expansion of services. This was probably not fully appreciated at that time because the importance of that report was primarily to show that past expenditure on the NHS was justified, rather than to explore how expenditure should be rationed.

In establishing the NHS, Aneurin Bevan's concern was to abolish rationing by price. In the month before the Appointed Day he said:

> If there is a shortage of doctors on 5 July, when the cash relationship between doctors and patients will disappear, it is very much more important that the doctors in short supply should spend their time looking after patients who really need to be looked after than that they should be looking after a lot of hypochondriacs who can afford to pay.[45]

It is unlikely that anyone would now disagree with the sentiment, but the problem remains of putting such rationing into practice. If we interpret rationing as the denial of access to some standard of care, disturbing features in the distortions of rationing before 1948 continued largely unchallenged for many years in the NHS. The advance of the vanguard identified by Foot was, if anything, enhanced by the NHS. Meanwhile, geographical inequalities persisted and the collective provision for the mentally handicapped, the mentally ill and the elderly (who often offer no promise of return by returning to or entering employment) was in some cases so inadequate that there were to be major scandals in certain hospitals.

The Delusion of Growth

The Persistence of Waiting Lists

Despite increases in staff, and more efficient use of resources, waiting lists are approximately as long now as they were in 1948, though there have been increases in number of patients treated. We began this chapter by describing the likely magnitude of sickness in the community, of which waiting lists are an imperfect measure. It would seem to be quite unrealistic to expect waiting lists to be removed by increases in supply (by extra resources and/or using current resources more efficiently). Referral rates by general practitioners are related in a complex way to hospital supply. Disputes and disruptive action by those who work in hospitals affect the delicate balance between arrival rate and service rate, with drastic consequences for lengths of waiting lists and waiting times (the astonishingly adverse results from minor reductions in service capacity are predictable from queueing theory). It is possible to make a short-term impact on the dramatic deterioration in service by more intensive work to remove the longer-than-average waiting times. It would however seem Utopian to expect to make a long-term impact on waiting lists by extra resources. And waiting lists, although often seen as a subject of concern, may be the fairest way of rationing treatment.

Resource Allocation to the Vanguard

One of the most fundamental distortions arising from the delusion of growth is the belief that what the vanguard enjoys today, can become universal tomorrow. Foot referred directly to the vanguard of British medicine — the best of the voluntary hospitals. At the inception of the NHS, in England and Wales, these were singled out for special treatment as teaching hospitals. They were to be administered by Boards of Governors with direct access to the Ministry — other hospitals were to be administered by Hospital Management Committees (HMCs) which were accountable via Regional Hospital Boards (RHBs) to the Ministry. Teaching hospitals were allowed to retain their trust funds to be used by their Boards of Governors at their discretion — all other hospitals had their funds pooled to be redistributed to hospitals according to size.

The Guillebaud Committee considered one of the major suggestions put to them that 'the service would be administered more economically and efficiently if the RHBs in England and Wales were made responsible for the teaching as well as the non-teaching hospitals in their Regions'.[46] The committee reviewed the arguments. The main report concluded that a convincing case had not been made for this change, which was rejected because 'one of the dangers of a national hospital system lies in overstandardisation and uniformity. There is a distinct advantage therefore in preserving the separate status of the teaching hospitals outside the Regional Hospital Board framework.'[47] Miss (later Dame) Anne

Godwin dissented from this majority view on three grounds. First, because she gained 'the impression . . . that the teaching hospitals, in their comparative isolation, have not been so acutely aware of the need for economies and the means of securing them as non-teaching hospitals'.[48] Second, and more important, that there is no obligation to harmonise development plans of the teaching hospital(s) and the RHB within which it (or they) are located. Third, that the pull on staff exercised by the prestige of teaching hospitals was enhanced by their isolation and would contribute to the maintenance of two standards within the NHS.

In 1973 Forsyth reviewed the position of teaching hospitals.[49] He pointed out that they accounted for five per cent of all hospitals and 6 per cent of all hospital beds, yet spent 14 per cent of all current expenditure on hospital services and 20 per cent of hospital capital expenditure. He suggested then that the inequitable distribution of skills and resources to teaching hospitals was due to their separate administration and closer access to the DHSS. In 1976 David Owen suggested that part of the reason why expenditure on teaching hospitals rose proportionately more than expenditure on general hospitals in the 1960s was that the former are in the forefront of technological innovation and scientific medicine.[50] On reorganisation in 1974 the special status ended for undergraduate teaching hospitals, most of which are now being squeezed under current policies of moving towards a more equitable allocation of services in England. But in 1976 Dr Owen suggested that the teaching hospitals' large share of capital expenditure (20 per cent) was often not related to service needs.[51]

We pursue the difficult problems of equity in resource allocation in Chapter 8. What is relevant here is why teaching hospitals were allowed to perpetuate the dual standards suspected by Anne Godwin in 1956, confirmed by Forsyth in 1973 and by the DHSS Resource Allocation Working Party in 1976. The special administrative arrangements may have helped initially but do not of themselves constitute an adequate explanation. They could equally well have served to reverse earlier policies of overgenerous funding of teaching hospitals. Nor can we merely rest on explanations that teaching hospitals contained the most influential members of the medical profession, unless we can understand why they were able to exercise this influence. In Chapter 1 we suggested that the failure to examine critically hospital procedures is consistent with a yearning for belief in the power of medicine when we are sick. Later in this chapter we suggest that the alleged medical bias against improvements in long-stay care may well be one shared by the community at large. The preferential funding of teaching hospitals can be seen as consistent with a general aspiration to promote health care of the highest standards. The maintenance of the vanguard in which doctors are trained accords with a hope of a better future.

The Real Increases in Staff and Services

In this section we identify how the increases in NHS resources at constant prices were translated into service development. In the following two sections we explore how these increases were distributed geographically, and which services were neglected. Figure 1.1 of Chapter 1 shows that the steady growth of the NHS at constant prices began in 1954. Table 2.1 gives a breakdown of this expenditure for 1956–7 and 1976–7.

Table 2.1: The Pattern of Growth in NHS Expenditure in England and Wales (at November 1976 Prices)

Item	1956–7		1976–7		Increase	
Health Authorities:	£m	%	£m	%	£m	% share of total increase
Current	2,167	68	3,773	70	1,606	73
Capital	55	2	423	8	368	17
Family Practitioner Services	979	30	1,182	22	216	10
Totals	3201	100	5,378	100	2,177	100

Source: Annual Report of the DHSS for 1977, Cmnd 7394, p. 35.

Of the increase of over £2,000m in the 20-year period, 90 per cent was accounted for by expenditure by Health Authorities, and 73 per cent took the form of increases in their current expenditure. Table 2.2 gives the Government's statement of planned expenditure for 1982–3. This shows trends from 1976–7, as planned in January 1979.

The most striking feature of planned development of the NHS is that less will be spent in real terms on *capital* work in 1982–3 than in 1976–7 – see Figure 2.1; the peak of capital expenditure was reached in 1973. The family practitioner services show a substantial increase, mainly because of the growth in the drug bill. *Current* expenditure by Health Authorities and Boards is planned to continue to consume 70 per cent of NHS expenditure. Table 2.3 uses provisional figures for

Figure 2.1: Health Programmes — UK (At 1978 Survey Prices. Excludes Personal Social Services)

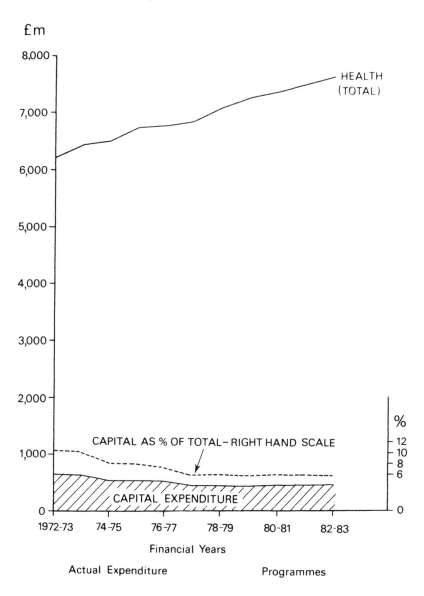

Source: See Table 3 of Appendix.

Table 2.2: Planned Growth in NHS Expenditure for Great Britain (at November 1977 Prices)

Item	1976–77 £m	%	1982–83 £m	%	Increase £m	% share in total increase
Health Authorities etc.						
Hospitals and Community Health Services						
Current	4,525	70	5,108	71	583	77
Capital	495	8	433	6	–62	–8
Family Practitioner Services	1,395	22	1,633	23	238	31
Totals	6,415	100	7,174	100	759	100

Source: *The Government's Expenditure Plans 1979–80 to 1982–83,* Cmnd 7439 (HMSO, London, 1979), Table 2.11 and see also p. 145 for details of FPS expenditure in certain years. Other health services are omitted.

1977–8 for current expenditure in England to break down the total (of £3,931m) for hospitals and community services.

Table 2.3: Distribution of Revenue Expenditure — Hospital and Community Health Services only (England, 1977–8)

	%	
Salaries and wages:		
Medical and dental	8.8	
Nursing	31.0	
Professional etc.	6.8	
Administrative and clerical	9.3	
Ancillary and ambulance	18.4	
		74.3
Other costs:		
Drugs and dressings	3.5	
Medical and surgical equipment, etc.	5.6	
Heat, light and power	3.5	
Estate maintenance	2.6	
Other (net of charges to staff etc.)	10.5	
		25.7
Total net expenditure		100.0

Source: DHSS (provisional figures).

Nearly 75 per cent of current expenditure by Health Authorities in 1977–8 was on wages and salaries. This means that whenever we talk about savings in current expenditure these almost invariably entail redeploying or sacking staff.

Table 2.4 analyses increases in hospital staffing from the early years of the NHS to its reorganisation in 1974. Table 2.5 compares growth from before reorganisation to 1977, for England alone.

Table 2.4: Growth in Hospital Staff Numbers in England and Wales 1949 to 1974*

			Increase	
	1949	1974	Numbers	% of 1949
Medical	11,735	27,057	15,322	130
Dental	206	835	629	305
Regional Hospital Board Headquarters staff	1,320	8,533	7,213	646
Nursing	137,636	321,249	183,613	133
Midwifery	9,043	18,211	9,168	101
Hospital professional and Technical	13,940	39,944	26,004	186
Hospital administrative and clerical	23,797	60,745	36,948	155
Ancillary, maintenance etc.	157,112	239,735	82,623	52
Total	354,789	716,309	361,520	102

Sources: *Compendium of Health Statistics* (2nd ed Office of Health Economics, 1977), Table 2.1; supplemented by Health and Personal Social Services Statistics for Wales, no. 3 (HMSO, Cardiff, 1976) (for Welsh Hospital Board Headquarters Staff for 1974).

*There are a number of definitional changes which mean that some of these figures are not strictly comparable.

Until reorganisation the increases in staff expenditure arose mainly from the increased number of nursing and ancillary staff, even though the proportionate increases in their numbers were low in comparison with those of other staff. Since reorganisation the increase in numbers has been greatest in the nursing group, though the largest proportionate increase has been in administrative and clerical staff. That increase has been stopped by the demand for reductions in management. We can gain some appreciation of the direction in growth of staffing of those concerned directly with the treatment of patients by examining the

Table 2.5: Growth in Hospital Staff Numbers in England, 1973 to 1977

Staff Description	Whole-time Equivalent		Increase	
	1973	1977	Numbers	% of 1973
Medical	27,354	31,131	3,777	13
Dental	2,216	2,361	145	6
RHA HQ, etc.[1]	10.590	12,640	2,050	19
Nursing	284,068	319,756	35,688	12
Midwifery	19,426	20,056	630	3
Professional and Technical[2]	44,155	52,798	8,643	19
Works and maintenance	19,550	23,059	3,509	18
Administrative and clerical[3]	68,846	88,819	19,973	29
Ambulance staff	16,594	17,383	789	5
Ancillary and others	163,886	171,465	7,579	5
Total (Regional and Area Health Authorities and Boards of Governors staff)	656,685	739,468	82,783	13

1 Include RHA headquarters, mass radiography, blood transfusion service and other regional unit staff.
2 Includes 2,349 hospital social workers for 1973 — responsibility for these staff was transferred to Local Authority Social Services on 1 April 1974.
3 The 1973 figure includes Former Executive Council Staff.

growth in consultant appointments. Table 2.6 gives the growth from 1950 in the total number of consultants and the ten specialties with the most numerous complements in 1977.

These figures indicate a shift in emphasis in medical treatment: the three specialties with the greatest number of consultants in 1950 were general surgery, general medicine and anaesthetics respectively; in 1978 anaesthetics, mental health and pathology had become the three specialties with the most consultants. Mental health together with the supporting specialties of anaesthetics and pathology account for 33 per cent of the total increase in consultant appointments. Unfortunately supply has not grown to meet demand for these posts. The 1979 planning circular issued by the DHSS[52] told Health Authorities to plan on the basis that shortages of trained candidates would continue to constrain the number of new posts which could be approved in psychiatry, anaesthetics and pathology. (There are also serious constraints in radiology and geriatric medicine.)

We can relate the increase of over 100 per cent in hospital staffing (from some 350,000 in 1949 to over 700,000 in 1974) to the number

Table 2.6: Growth in Consultant Strength in England and Wales

Description	Consultant Strength						Increase	
	1950[1]			1978[2]				% of total
'Top Ten' by Specialty	No.	%		No.	%		Numbers	increase
Anaesthetics	554	10		1,563	12		1,009	14
Mental	454	8		1,522	12		1,068	15
Pathology	487	8		1,436	11		949	14
General Medicine	717	12		1,063	8		346	5
General Surgery	811	14		945	7		134	2
Radiology	340	6		783	6		443	6
Orthopaedic Surgery	242	4		624	5		382	5
Obstetrics and Gynacology	381	7		698	5		317	5
Paediatrics	175	3		469	4		294	4
Dentistry	236	4		481	4		245	4
Total 'Top Ten'	4,397	76		9,584	75		5,187	74
Total All Specialties	5,781	100		12,766	100		6,985	100

Sources: 1 Report of Ministry of Health, 1 April 1950 to 31 December 1951, Cmd 8655 (HMSO).
2 DHSS.

of patients treated, which increased by 67 per cent (from just under three million to just over five million). The increase in staff concerned directly with health care (medical, dental, midwifery and nursing) was of nearly 132 per cent (from nearly 160,000 to nearly 370,000), and the increase over the 25 years in staff input per patient treated works out at over a third. This, of course, does not by itself mean a decrease in efficiency because the data only relate to *throughput,* the passage of patients through hospital, and not to *output,* the improvement in patients' conditions. In part the decline in this crude measure of productivity is due to shorter working hours. If we take account of developments in medicine (indicated by the growth in consultant strength of anaesthetists and pathologists), increases in staffing may well be explicable in terms of the increased workload and the decline in the number of hours in the working week.

Whilst staffing levels have increased faster than patient throughput there has been a decline in the number of available hospital beds. The throughput per bed has increased from 6.6 in 1949 to 14.2 in 1977, and the length of stay in hospital for specialties excluding geriatric and psychiatric has declined from 18.9 days in 1953 to 9.2 in 1977. The trend for the reductions for length of stay in the average now seems to be flattening out, although there may be scope for further reductions by developments in day care, domiciliary care and intensive out-patient treatment. This raises, however, the contentious issue of balancing institutional and community care (which we touch on in Chapter 9). And there appear to be problems in continuing to increase bed-occupancy rates: pressure on beds might contribute, for example, to inter-personal tensions and even to disruptive behaviour.

Geographical Inequality in the Provision of Health Care

Following the publication of the Beveridge Report in 1942 the Coalition Government presented in 1944 a White Paper on *A National Health Service.*[53] This reviewed current arrangements and highlighted inequality in access to medical treatment. It stated that whether people could get the services they require still depended 'too much upon circumstance, upon where they happen to live or work, to what group (e.g. of age or vocation) they happen to belong, or what happens to be the matter with them'.[54] One of the intentions of the National Health Service was 'To ensure that everybody in the country — irrespective of means, age, sex or occupation — should have equal opportunity to benefit from the best and most up-to-date medical and allied services available.'[55] The Treasury had been concerned about this intention in the draft of the White Paper, but their objections about promising geographical equity were not upheld.[56] This matter was taken up at Permanent Secretary level when Sir Bernard Gilbert (Treasury) commented on the galleys of the White Paper in a letter to Sir John Maude (Ministry of Health) as follows:

> . . . in galley 3 you spoke of people's ability to get medical and allied services as depending too much on where they happen to live. I imagine that by this you mean whether they happen to live in a backward or a forward area, but is it not possible that the reader may think that you are not going to overcome the differences in local enterprise but in geographical situation. I do not suppose that anybody would imagine that the man who lives in the Outer Hebrides could be as well served as the man who lives next door to a London hospital, but there are many intermediate cases, and we should have thought it would be wise to have a qualifying phrase in your report as a safeguard against the formation of excessive expectations.[57]

The qualifying phrase asked for by Sir Bernard Gilbert was not included. In 1945 the Minister of Health of the newly elected Labour Government, Aneurin Bevan, in a draft Cabinet Paper[58] rejected local government administration of the NHS because there would tend to be 'a better service in the richer areas, a worse service in the poorer'. The aim of the NHS was 'to achieve as nearly as possible a uniform standard of service for all'. This was particularly important since everyone would be paying the same national rates and would therefore expect 'an equally good service' to be available everywhere.[59]

The Treasury comments on this draft agreed that 'with purely central finance, it would not be possible to defend any material divergence in the standard of service as between one area and another'[60] and that complete uniformity would not be achieved under local government. Two of the concerns of the Treasury were that whilst a nationalised service would be more efficient, it would also be more expensive,[61] and that financing the current inequalities by taxes rather than by rates would give greater benefit to the rich, because the highest hospital expenditure was found in the richest areas.[62]

In 1976, nearly thirty years after the inception of a centrally financed and administered National Health Service, an official working party (the Resource Allocation Working Party — RAWP) of the Department of Health and Social Security described the methods used to distribute financial resources to the NHS since its inception as tending to perpetuate the historic situation.[63] These methods allocated revenue on the basis of past allocations plus an increment plus extra revenue to cover the running cost of completed capital projects (the Revenue Consequences of Capital Schemes). The RAWP saw this last element as distorting capital development: 'its important characteristic as an investment for the future has been sacrificed in the interests of preserving consumption at a particular level'.[64] The report criticised geographical inequalities in the quantity, age and condition of available capital stock; its distribution was still 'influenced by historic patterns of health care delivery'.[65]

In the early 1950s, we have seen that it had been expected that expenditure on health care would be self-limiting, and continued increases in expenditure were attributed to maladministration and inefficiency. As long as the Ministry expected expenditure to be self-limiting there would be less need to be concerned about inequalities: in time, as extra resources became available, a uniform standard could be achieved. The Guillebaud Committee concluded that expenditure would be open-ended. But for much of the post-war period, questions of distribution were not generally seen as significant issues. The dominant ideology was much more concerned with 'making the cake bigger' rather than the distribution of the national cake.

From the inception of the NHS, the Government had been rationing resources for health care, but the first response was perhaps to ration according to demand as expressed by the various responsible hospital boards, who would think in terms of present and prospective demand for their services. The RAWP report emphasised the importance of distinguishing between demand and need. This is a particularly important distinction in resource allocation because there is ample evidence to show that supply fuels demand. Thus allocating incrementally on the basis of past allocations – i.e. on the basis of supply – can also appear to be rationing according to demand.

By the late 1960s distribution was becoming an issue. Crossman describes in his diary in 1969, when he was Secretary for Health and Social Services, a paper describing revenue allocations to hospitals. He says that these allocations favoured the London hospitals 'with great unfairness to Sheffield, Newcastle and Birmingham, which are greatly under-financed'.[66] In 1970 a new formula was introduced to reduce inequality. Crossman describes his meeting with Regional Hospital Board Chairmen when he discussed this formula; he says that there was a tremendous struggle to maintain the status quo.[67]

In terms of expenditure per head, the regional inequalities in revenue have been reduced: in the mid-1960s there was a spread of over 50 per cent around the national average in terms of population; by 1976–7 this spread had been reduced to 36 per cent.[68] In capital in England the spread of provision around the national average was about 50 per cent in 1948 and was the same 25 years later.[69] In Chapter 8 we review current policies on moving towards a more equitable allocation of resources in England.

Inequalities in Service Development

A report published in 1978 described conditions at Normansfield Hospital for the Mentally Handicapped: 'With one exception . . . the wards were bare and . . . reminiscent of scenes from a workhouse of old.'[70] And another witness, describing Normansfield, said, 'It was just as if Dickens had come alive again in the mid-1970s in the middle of Teddington.'[71] The harsh conditions of the Dickensian workhouse – but not those said to resemble them in this NHS hospital – were explicitly designed to discourage the able-bodied unemployed from seeking the relief the workhouses provided. These Poor Law principles were laid down in 1834 but the Royal Commission of that year recommended separate workhouses for the sick so that they should not be subjected to the same conditions as those intended to encourage the able-bodied to find employment. Unfortunately this recommendation was not fully implemented, and the scandalous existence of providing the same workhouse for the sick and the able-bodied was condemned by the Majority and Minority Reports of the 1904–9 Royal Commission into the Poor Law, and by Neville Chamberlain in a speech in the House of Commons as late as 1928.[72] At the inception of the NHS the remaining Poor Law institutions caring for the sick were taken into the regional structure. Hospitals were to be administered by officers who were accountable to Hospital Management Committees (HMCs) and to Regional Hospital Boards (RHBs). In many cases the buildings remained the same, being adapted to the extent that funds permitted. Twenty years later the first of a series of official reports were published which caused concern about conditions in certain hospitals providing long-stay care. We mention some of these: it will, however, be clear that inadequacy of service often came from poor local management rather than from central policies or allocations.

A White Paper published in 1968 criticised the management of certain geriatric and psychiatric hospitals, and other distressing reports appeared on hospitals for the mentally ill and the mentally handicapped.[73] These again were critical of management, the HMCs and the

RHBs. The Ely Inquiry of 1969 criticised the tripartite administrative structure of the NHS.[74] The RHB (the Welsh Hospital Board) and its officers were criticised for not accepting responsibility for the inspection or supervision of standards and not using their powers to bring about any improvement. In making recommendations the report identified overriding objectives which could only be achieved if substantially increased financial resources were made available, and asked for a critical review and overhaul of the organisation and administration of the HMC. The 1971 *Report of the Farleigh Hospital Committee of Inquiry*[75] stated as its first principal conclusion that the RHB and the HMC had paid far too little attention to the patients at the hospital and had failed to recognise national trends in the care of mentally handicapped adults. It recommended that RHBs should intensify their reviews of the level of expenditure and staffing in hospitals for the mentally handicapped. The 1972 *Report of the Committee of Inquiry into Whittingham Hospital* concluded that 'The management structure has not proved equal to its task.'[76] Its recommendation that the members of the HMC be invited to resign and the committee reconstituted was implemented. It criticised the Manchester Regional Hospital Board for failing to recognise the problems of implementing their programme of reorganising services for the mentally ill.

Following the Ely Hospital Report the Hospital Advisory Service (HAS – later Health Advisory Service) was introduced. (This at first concentrated on conditions in long-stay hospitals but its remit has been extended and now covers health and personal social services.) In 1971 the Government published *Better Services for the Mentally Handicapped.*[77] In 1974 the NHS was reorganised to overcome weaknesses in the tripartite structure of 1948. In 1978 the *Report of the Committee of Inquiry into Normansfield Hospital* gave amongst its principal conclusions:

The main cause for the shortfall in patient care and development was not lack of finance but a failure of duty by the Area Health Authority (and in particular the Area Management Team). The Regional Health Authority failed adequately to monitor the work of the Area Health Authority and did not ensure that its policy in relation to the delivery of care to the mentally handicapped was carried out. There was a significant failure to implement the policy laid down in the Government White Paper *Better Services for the Mentally Handicapped.*[78]

The reorganisation had not overcome the problems of lack of leadership – the report on Normansfield identified similar problems to those of Ely. The Hospital Advisory Service had made two critical reports on Normansfield in 1970 and 1972. The remedial action which began following the 1970 report ran into difficulties because of lack of finance and changed fire-safety standards. Intentions to act on the 1972 report appear to have been dissipated by the impending reorganisation. The report on Normansfield identified a sense of despair, and belief in the lack of adequate machinery to deal with the problems of the hospital. It rejects these attitudes: 'Health Authorities have a right and indeed a duty, to stipulate, if they feel it necessary, the pattern of life that they wish to provide in the hospitals for which they are responsible (this particularly applies to long-stay hospitals).'[79]

Long-stay care is sometimes inappositely described as the 'Cinderella' services. Whilst the Cinderella of the fairy tale was neglected, her rivals were ugly sisters, and the story ends happily because her beauty is recognised by Prince Charming following one timely intervention by her fairy godmother. The report on Normansfield referred to the difficulties of caring for 'the helpless, many of whom are doubly incontinent and more or less irrational all of the time'.[80] The staff had to ' "gather and tend the fragments that yet remain" of grossly mentally and physically handicapped people'.[81] The image of a beautiful young woman is an inappropriate motif for the plight of such patients. A number of policy interventions have been attempted but it seems that progress depends on continuous effort by those responsible, whose dedicated efforts are too little appreciated. The Prince Charming who provides the means for such progress is the taxpayer. Increasingly, the heavy staff costs required by the altruism of caring for the mentally handicapped can only be financed by forgoing developments in acute care. Long-stay care was neglected during a much easier economic climate than is now in prospect. Before 1948 long-stay care had been mainly the responsibility of local authorities. The 1948 arrangements evidently did not in all cases result in sufficient attention and sufficient funding by the RHBs; Government funds were allocated to each Board, but the disposal between acute and long-stay cases was left entirely to them. We review in Chapter 9 the problems of reversing the historic and continuing neglect of these services.

Doctors and Management of the NHS

It is vital to involve clinicians in the difficult problems of rationing resources for health care. If this rationing – or indeed the development

– of health resources is to be accomplished in the best interests of prospective patients, there need to be links between an epidemiological survey of the needs of the community, referrals by general practitioners, and service provided by hospital clinicians. The tripartite structure of 1948 was seen as hindering these links: a departmental report of 1972[82] (see below) was concerned about the failure of hospital doctors to involve general practitioners and Medical Officers of Health (employed by local authorities) in their committees. These weaknesses were to be remedied on reorganisation by new posts in community medicine at each level of the reorganised NHS and at district level (that typically organised around a District General Hospital) a new committee – the District Medical Committee – was to be established. This included the community physician, hospital-based doctors and general practitioners. However a departmental report[83] issued in the shadow of the impending reorganisation recorded misgivings amongst doctors about these innovations – although the report disagreed: 'Some consultants regard the role of the district community physician with suspicion, and fear that his part in helping to determine priorities will bring him into conflict with consensus views reached among clinicians',[84] and 'Some doctors . . . have questioned whether the district medical committee has a useful part to play in the new management arrangements.'[85] One of the most serious causes of concern about the reorganised NHS is that these innovations have indeed not fulfilled their promise. Some understanding of these disappointing outcomes can be gained from the different status and interests of the doctors intended to work together following reorganisation.

Community Medicine

Doctors expected to play a significant role in medical discussions in the reorganised NHS were trained in the 1960s or before. The *Report of the Royal Commission on Medical Education 1965–68* (the Todd Report) described recruitment of doctors to community medicine as 'unsatisfactory: most young doctors seek careers in clinical medicine',[86] and recommended a number of changes so that trainees in community medicine should see that it offers prospects 'clearly as good as those in other specialties'.[87]

A year earlier, a departmental report had commented on inadequate training of medical administrators for community medicine:

At present there is a regrettable lack of properly organised vocational training for professional medical administrators other than those required by local authorities. Until this is remedied and there is some improvement in the career structure, the present shortage of suitable applicants for this type of work seems likely to continue. . . There has been systematic training in the Diploma in Public Health for nearly a century, but this Diploma has been related to one particular field of medicine and is not fitted to the requirements of the hospital service or general practice.[88]

On reorganisation jobs of considerable status were created for community physicians but there was a shortage of suitably qualified staff.

The Management of Work in Hospitals

Before 1948 there were two distinct and separate traditions of hospital administration. Local authority hospitals were administered by a medical superintendent, who normally combined clinical and administrative duties. In voluntary hospitals (of which the teaching hospitals were the most distinguished) administrative responsibility was vested in the medical committee, which was responsible to the Board of Governors, but day-to-day administration was in the hands of the house governor. After 1948 long-stay hospitals tended to be administered by medical superintendents but general hospitals normally followed the model of the voluntary hospitals in England and Wales. In Scotland the traditional role of the medical superintendent continued after 1948.

The 1954 *Report on the Internal Administration of Hospitals* (the Bradbeer Report) rejected both these traditional arrangements: 'An alternative — applicable, we believe, in most of the larger general hospitals — is to appoint as medical administrator one of the consultants who has the talent, the taste and the time for this kind of work.'[89] Although that report was wholeheartedly endorsed by the Guillebaud Committee,[90] which was particularly concerned about the weak administrative links between hospital services and general practice and local authority services, it was not referred to by the first 'Cogwheel' Report of 1967[91] (see below). Perhaps of those consultants who had the talent for administration, few had the taste.

Two reports on the organisation of medical work in hospitals were published on the same day in 1967: the Godber Report[92] for England and Wales (known as the 'Cogwheel' Report from the device on its cover) and the Brotherston Report[93] for Scotland. Each advocated similar principles of organising medical staffs into groups of specialties (or one speciality), known as Divisions, where they provided a common service with the same call on resources. These divisions would have representatives (the Chairman of each division in Scotland) on an Executive Committee. In England and Wales the Chairman of this Medical Executive Committee was expected to be relieved of some of his clinical duties so that he could be a part-time administrator. In Scotland the working party did not envisage a major administrative role for his equivalent because of the continuing position of the medical superintendent in Scottish hospitals.

One of the continuing concerns of the Cogwheel Reports was the lack of co-ordination of care both within the hospital system and between hospitals, general practice and local authority services. The first report described the links as 'tenuous', which was reflected 'not only in the organisation of care for the individual but in the planning of care for the community as a whole'.[94]

In the light of developments recommended for the reorganised NHS, two observations made by the first Cogwheel Report are worth noting. First, whilst the working party was in no doubt that radical changes were needed in the organisation of medical work, it saw that the process of change 'must be the outcome of local consideration and conviction rather than the imposition of detailed methods arbitrarily defined centrally.'[95]

Few would see value in the imposition of methods determined arbitrarily. The important point is whether methods determined centrally appear to be arbitrary to hospitals and doctors who have to follow central guidance. This point was emphasised by the second Cogwheel Report in its misquotation of the above statement which, when reiterated, had the later part rephrased as 'imposition of detailed methods *centrally* defined'.[96] The reorganised NHS did impose statutory committees and clinical membership, but these do not seem adequate — unless determinedly operated by strong personalities — to resolve the difficult problems now facing the authorities. This point is amplified in Chapters 5 and 9.

The second observation of the first Cogwheel Report relevant to the reorganised NHS is its description of the extant advisory machinery, which was

> designed . . . to ensure the representation of the whole consultant and specialist medical and dental staff of the hospitals concerned, of general medical and dental practitioners on the staff and of those in practice in the area and of medical officers of health . . . such a committee, while democratic, is cumbersome and unwieldy for the manifold duties it has to carry out, ranging from major policy

considerations to more routine medical matters affecting possibly only one or two specialties.[97]

Similar criticisms were to be made of the new advisory committees established in the reorganised NHS.

The second Cogwheel Report reviewed the developments in the four years following the first report, and noted that its recommendations had been largely followed by the general hospitals for which the structure had been designed: almost two-thirds had established a divisional structure and just under a half had established a medical executive committee. The report lamented the lack of progress in the involvement of doctors from general practice and from local authorities:

> many matters decided in Cogwheel divisions and committees concern general practitioners and other doctors working in the community, whose representation at Cogwheel can do much to improve communication and in some matters lead to better decisions. We are disappointed that such representation (which appears to be confined to about one-third of Cogwheel structures) is so limited.[98]

We have already referred to the third Cogwheel Report and its comments in favour of the District Medical Committee (DMC) and community physicians. The DMC would represent all branches of the medical profession, and that report believed that 'only such a committee . . . can bring a truly integrated approach to wider aspects of hospital care'.[99] It could not, because it was too widely-based, perform the tasks of the Cogwheel structure, and this report saw the need for both Cogwheel and the new committees. It recognised that 'It will be even more important in future to guard against any unnecessary overlap of machinery or duplication of activity, so that the time of clinicians may be put to best use.'[100] The first Cogwheel Report criticised the existence of only one committee for all medical matters. Following the reorganisation there has been a proliferation of medical committees, with some confusion as to which is the appropriate committee for the formulation of medical advice.

Notes

1. Marjorie Tew, '"What Do Hospitals Do?", the Provision and Utilisation of Services in National Health Hospitals in England and Wales 1949–1973', Health Services Research Group Report No. 9 (University of Nottingham, 1975).

2. Ibid.
3. J.M. Last, 'The Iceberg', *Lancet*, vol. ii, 28 (1963).
4. British Medical Association, *Primary Medical Care*, Planning Report No. 4, 1970.
5. R.G.S. Brown, *The Changing National Health Service* (Routledge and Kegan Paul, London, 1973), p. 21.
6. Ibid.
7. A.R. Bradwell, M.H.B. Carnalt and T.P. Whitehead, 'Explaining the Unexpected Abnormal Results of Biochemical Profile Investigations', *Lancet*, vol. ii, 1071 (1974).
8. See W.P.D. Logan and E.M. Brooke, *The Survey of Sickness 1943–1952*, General Register Office Studies on Medical and Population Subjects No. 12 (HMSO, London, 1957).
9. Office of Population Censuses and Surveys, *General Household Survey 1976* (HMSO, London, 1978), Table 8.1.
10. Ibid., p. 72.
11. Department of Health and Social Security (DHSS), *The Way Forward* (HMSO, London, 1977), p. 3.
12. David Owen, *In Sickness and In Health, The Politics of Medicine* (Quartet, London, 1976), p. 54.
13. DHSS, *Sharing Resources for Health in England*, Report of the Resource Allocation Working Party (the RAWP Report) (HMSO, London, 1976), p. 7.
14. DHSS, *Priorities for Health and Personal Social Services in England*, A Consultative Document (HMSO, London, 1976).
15. Scottish Home and Health Department (SHHD), *Scottish Health Authorities Revenue Equalisation (SHARE)* (HMSO, Edinburgh, 1977).
16. RAWP Report.
17. SHHD. *Revenue Equalisation*, p. 3.
18. R.G.S. Brown, *Reorganising the National Health Service, A Case Study of Administrative Change* (Basil Blackwell and Martin Robertson, Oxford, 1979).
19. Sir William Beveridge, *Social Insurance and Allied Services* (the Beveridge Report), Cmd 6404 (HMSO, London, 1942), p. 5.
20. Ibid., p. 17.
21. Ibid., p. 105.
22. *Report on the Future Provision of Medical and Allied Services* (the Dawson Report), Cmd 693 (HMSO, London, 1920).
23 Michael Foot, *Aneurin Bevan, 1945–1960* (Paladin, London, 1975), p. 209.
24. Ibid., p. 210.
25. Ibid., p. 250.
26. Public Records Office, Treasury T161/1166, S50599.
27. Foot, *Aneurin Bevan*, p. 250.
28. House of Commons Debates, 10 February 1949, col. 536.
29. Ibid., 14 March 1950, col. 916.
30. Ffrangcon Roberts, *The Cost of Health* (Turnstile Press, London, 1952).
31. *Report of the Committee of Enquiry into the Cost of the National Health Service* (the Guillebaud Report), Cmd 9663 (HMSO, London, 1956), p.1.
32. Brian Abel-Smith and R.M. Titmuss, *The Cost of the National Health Service* (Cambridge University Press, 1956).
33. Guillebaud Report, p. 268.
34. Ibid., p. 269.
35. Ibid., p. 50.
36. Ibid.
37. Foot, *Aneurin Bevan*, p. 101.
38. Ibid., p. 102.

39. Ibid., p. 103.

40. National Insurance Act, 1911.

41. See Gordon Forsyth, *Doctors and State Medicine* (Pitman, London, 1973), pp. 19–20.

42. Beveridge Report, p. 167.

43. Guillebaud Report, p. 50.

44. DHSS, *The Way Forward*, p. 28.

45. Foot, *Aneurin Bevan*, p. 209.

46. Guillebaud Report, p. 72.

47. Ibid., p. 75.

48. Ibid., p. 270.

49. Forsyth, *Doctors and State Medicine*, pp. 127–9.

50. Owen, *In Sickness and In Health*, p. 53.

51. Ibid., p. 74.

52. DHSS, *Health Service Development, Health and Personal Social Services In England, DHSS Planning Guidelines for 1979/80*, Health Circular HC (79)9(1979).

53. *A National Health Service*, Cmd 6502 (HMSO, London, 1944).

54. Ibid., p. 6.

55. Ibid., p. 47.

56. Public Records Office, Treasury T161/1166, S50599.

57. Ibid.

58. Public Records Office, Treasury SS Division, 1242, S50599/06/1.

59. Ibid. Draft Cabinet Paper CP(45)13.

60. Ibid., Treasury minute of 15.12.45.

61. Ibid., Treasury minute of 6.10.45.

62. Ibid., Treasury minute of 6.3.46.

63. RAWP Report, p. 7.

64. Ibid., p. 10.

65. Ibid.

66. Richard Crossman. *The Diaries of a Cabinet Minister, Volume Three* (Hamish Hamilton and Jonathan Cape, London, 1977), p. 569.

67. Ibid., p. 876.

68. Owen, *In Sickness and In Health*, p. 49.

69. Ibid., p. 48.

70. *Report of the Committee of Inquiry into Normansfield Hospital*, Cmnd 7357 (HMSO, London, 1978), p. 15.

71. Ibid., p. 27.

72. See Brian Watkin, *Documents on Health and Social Services, 1834 to the Present Day* (Methuen, London, 1975), pp. 1–31 for a concise review of Poor Law reports and legislation.

73. *Findings and Recommendations Following Enquiries into Allegations Concerning the Care of Elderly Patients in Certain Hospitals*, Cmnd 3687 (HMSO, London, 1968), pp. 21–53.

74. *Report of the Committee of Inquiry into Allegations of Ill-Treatment of Patients, and Other Irregularities at the Ely Hospital, Cardiff*, Cmnd 3975 (HMSO, London, 1969).

75. *Report of the Farleigh Hospital Committee of Inquiry*, Cmnd 4557 (HMSO, London, 1971).

76. *Report of the Committee of Inquiry into Whittingham Hospital*, Cmnd 4861 (HMSO, London, 1972), p. 40.

77. DHSS, *Better Services for the Mentally Handicapped*, Cmnd 4683 (HMSO, London, 1971).

78. *Normansfield Report*, p. 9.

79. Ibid., p. 407.

80. Ibid., p. 2.

81. Ibid.

82. DHSS, *Second Report of the Joint Working Party on the Organisation of Medical Work in Hospitals* (second Cogwheel Report) (HMSO, London, 1972).

83. DHSS, *Third Report of the Joint Working Party on the Organisation of Medical Work in Hospitals* (third Cogwheel Report) (HMSO, London, 1974).

84. Ibid., p. 23.

85. Ibid., p. 17.

86. *Report of the Royal Commission on Medical Education 1965–68* (Todd Report) (HMSO, London, 1968), p. 67.

87. Ibid.

88. Ministry of Health, *First Report of the Joint Working Party on the Organisation of Medical Work in Hospitals* (first Cogwheel Report) (HMSO, London, 1967), p. 20.

89. Central Health Services Council, *Report of the Committee on the Internal Administration of Hospitals* (the Bradbeer Report) (HMSO, London, 1954), paras. 62–84.

90. Guillebaud Report, pp. 145–7.

91. First Cogwheel Report.

92. Ibid.

93. SHHD, *Organisation of Medical Work in the Hospital Service in Scotland,* First Report of the Joint Working Party (the Brotherston Report) (HMSO, Edinburgh, 1967).

94. First Cogwheel Report, p. 1.

95. Ibid., p. 3.

96. Second Cogwheel Report, p. 4.

97. First Cogwheel Report, p. 15.

98. Second Cogwheel Report, p. 15.

99. Third Cogwheel Report, p. 18.

100. Ibid., p. 7.

3 ORGANISATION AND MANAGEMENT

This chapter begins by summarising the form of organisation and management structure in the health services prior to the 1974 reorganisation. The post-1974 organisation and management structure is then explained.[1] Given that the organisational and management arrangements altered very substantially at reorganisation; that these alterations have affected communications, planning, resource allocation, financial control and working relationships generally within the health services; and that many of the alterations have apparently caused a great deal of critical reaction and resentment, it is important to have the main features of the 1974 reorganisation clearly in mind before considering the issues raised in later chapters. Our description and terminology applies to England, and generally to Wales: certain differences in Northern Ireland, Scotland and Wales are mentioned in a later section of the chapter.

NHS Organisation Prior to 1974

Between 1948 and 1974 the NHS operated under an organisation structure that largely retained and institutionalised the tripartite division of labour that had evolved during the century prior to the NHS being founded. The three divisions were the hospital services, the community and public health services provided by local government, and the family doctor and other practitioner services that had traditionally been conducted on an independent, 'self-employed' basis. Indeed one might almost describe the structure as fourfold, because within the hospital services the teaching hospitals enjoyed a substantial degree of independence from the remainder of the hospital system. The overall organisation structure prior to 1974 is summarised in Figure 3.1.

The hospital services were organised originally into fourteen, later fifteen, regions in England and Wales prior to 1974. Each region had its own Regional Hospital Board (RHB) and generally at least one medical school within its boundaries. The medical schools and associated teaching hospitals provided a focus for medical interest, research and regional-specialty services. Each RHB was directly responsible to the Minister of Health for the overall planning, provision and co-ordination of hospital and specialist services within its region.

Within each region there were typically twenty or more Hospital

Figure 3.1:   NHS Organisation Prior to 1974

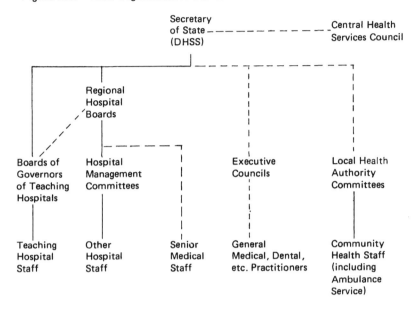

Key: Solid lines indicate direct responsibility.
       Broken lines indicate looser consultative, contractual and supervisory
       relationships.

Management Committees (HMCs) which were held responsible for the management of local groups of related (non-teaching) hospitals. Hospital staff were appointed on the authority of the HMCs, except that senior medical staff, of the status of Senior Registrar upwards, were appointed under contract to the RHBs (within guidelines and quotas of approved senior posts specified by the DHSS). Each HMC had considerable autonomy over the budgetary allocation of its revenue funds, but the approval of its RHB was required for major capital spending and for new specialty developments.

Teaching hospitals were administered by Boards of Governors directly responsible to the Secretary of State. However, one-fifth of the members of each Board of Governors were appointed by its RHB, and there was sufficient interaction amongst senior personnel on the Boards of Governors, within the medical schools and teaching hospitals, and at the RHB, to ensure some degree of co-ordination between the teaching hospitals and the mainstream hospital services.

The general medical, dental, ophthalmic and pharmaceutical services – the 'primary care' services – were administered by Executive Councils for the more than 100 areas that, insofar as practicable, matched up with local authority boundaries. Local Health Authorities held one-quarter of the seats on Executive Councils, to encourage co-ordination between primary care practitioners and community health care and personal social services. In practice, the Executive Councils had very limited authority to undertake health policy initiatives, and their main activity was to administer practitioners' contracts and remuneration – although they did additionally deal with complaints (other than complaints relating wholly to professional matters), and sometimes they had a role in influencing local developments such as the encouragement of primary care practitioners to work from health centres.

Community health services were provided, prior to reorganisation, by some 175 local Health Authorities. These were administered by the corresponding local government authorities, although the Secretary of State at the DHSS did have general supervisory influence on their activities. The community health services included the provision of antenatal and child health clinics, midwifery, health visiting and domiciliary nursing, family planning and health education, immunisation, services for the mentally ill and handicapped, ambulance services and certain other public health responsibilities.

NHS Management Prior to 1974

The last ten years prior to the NHS reorganisation in 1974 were marked by growing concern about the NHS and the need to alter the NHS in some way so as to achieve better integration of the separate 'compartments' of health care, and to redistribute health resources more equitably both as among the services and also geographically across the health regions and their local subdivisions. We have traced the development of these and other concerns in the preceding chapter, as part of the discussion of how the aspirations of and for the health services evolved through time. Nevertheless, and in spite of the gradual growth of trade union militancy and of the self-consciousness and assertiveness of various NHS professions (e.g. nurses and technicians), it seems fair to conclude that the operational-management environment in the NHS had not altered materially since the foundation of the NHS, or even earlier. That is, management activity was concentrated at the level of the individual hospital and its HMC, and at the local Health Authority offices. The hospital secretary was a person of established status who largely ran the hospital to meet the hospital consultants' perceptions of their needs for their patients. The hospital matron ran the nursing side with authority to achieve the same objective.

The typical HMC served a locality of fewer than 150,000 people. It was not remote. It was responsive to local medical opinion as to their perceived needs. Contact, or at least contentious contact, was limited between the HMC and its RHB. NHS funds and resources were growing from year to year, and the principle of 'incremental growth' of most health activities and locations – as opposed to more recent policies of selective growth and resource redistribution – meant that discussions with the RHB were largely concerned with new incremental developments, and their relative priorities and timing.

NHS Organisation After 1974

The reorganised NHS came into being on 1 April 1974. This followed several years of public debate based upon government papers, academic studies, and reports and proposals from professional and other pressure groups, and it was authorised by the National Health Service Reorganisation Act, 1973.[2] The local government reorganisation took place on the same date in 1974, which was convenient in view of the transfer of most local authority health services to the NHS, as this affected both reorganisations. In passing, it may be noted that although the local government reorganisation was arguably considerably less drastic than that required in the health services (in respect of the creation of extra levels of management structure, and of the attempt to integrate branches of services that previously had operated under quite independent and disparate management arrangements), in fact the Local Government Act, 1972, gave local authorities a longer time than health services to plan and arrange their organisational changeover. Local authorities were thus in a position to advertise their new appointments in advance of the NHS, so that they had first choice of the available job-seekers in respect of accountants, computer staff and certain management and other staff whose skills could be equally well applied in either local authorities or Health Authorities. Indeed, new NHS authorities created by reorganisation did not have time to complete filling appointments below their senior posts prior to the operative date of reorganisation, and of course in such circumstances only limited administrative arrangements for the new individual Health Authorities and Health Districts could be worked out in advance of the reorganisation date. Hence a considerable degree of confusion, and an otherwise unnecessary degree of damage to morale, occurred at the very inception of the new

NHS structure. The organisation structure of the NHS since 1974 is summarised in Figure 3.2.

Figure 3.2: NHS Organisation After 1974

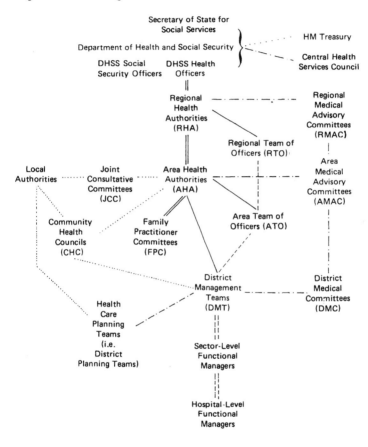

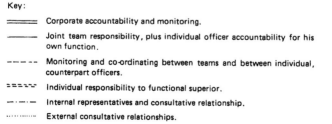

Key:

═════ Corporate accountability and monitoring.

─────── Joint team responsibility, plus individual officer accountability for his own function.

─ ─ ─ ─ Monitoring and co-ordinating between teams and between individual, counterpart officers.

≈≈≈≈≈ Individual responsibility to functional superior.

─ · ─ · ─ Internal representatives and consultative relationship.

············ External consultative relationships.

The Secretary of State and the DHSS

The Government published the so-called 'Grey Book' to explain, as its title indicates, the *Management Arrangements for the Reorganised National Health Service.*[3] The Grey Book specifies that the Secretary of State for Social Services, together with the DHSS, will be responsible for establishing national policies and priorities to determine the kind, scale and balance of NHS services.[4] They will review and approve Regional Health Authority (RHA) plans and allocate resources between RHAs.[5] The Secretary of State will be accountable for the performance of the NHS, and the DHSS will monitor RHA performance in relation to agreed objectives, and targets, including control over income and expenditure.[6] The Secretary of State will appoint RHA members and the chairmen of AHAs.[7] RHAs will be accountable to him and he will have powers of direction over them.[8] The DHSS will control the use of certain resources (e.g. remuneration and conditions of service, number and distribution of certain staff, and major building projects, etc.).[9]

The DHSS was created in 1968 by the merging of the two separate Ministries of Social Security and Health. The social security side of the DHSS was concerned mainly with administering the distribution of benefits and welfare provisions through local offices, whilst the health side of the DHSS continued its role of providing a headquarters administration for each separate part of the tripartite health services as then organised (i.e. hospital, primary and community services). However, the reorganisation of personal social services administration at the DHSS, together with the intention to reorganise the NHS, led to a review of the functions and organisation of the health side of the DHSS, effective at the end of 1972. Perhaps the most important developments were the creation of a Regional Group with regional liaison staff and other specialists to assist the planning and control of health services on a regional basis; together with the formation of a Service Development Group to study, plan for and promote the future development of the NHS in a manner to cut across the old tripartite boundaries, concentrating on patients' needs assessed by care group (i.e. children, the mentally handicapped, etc.).[10]

Personal social services other than health services are provided locally by metropolitan districts and non-metropolitan counties, subject to the general guidance of the Secretary of State at the DHSS. These services include child care, residential services for the elderly and the disabled, domiciliary services such as home helps, care of the handicapped, mental health services, social-work training, voluntary services liaison and care of the homeless. Within the DHSS a small staff section works with the Director of Social Services to assist planning and liaison for the co-ordination of health-service and social-service agencies, especially as regards the welfare of children, the elderly and the chronically sick and handicapped.

Regional Health Authorities

Upon reorganisation, fourteen RHAs took over from the former Regional Hospital Boards in England, although with some boundary alterations so that each RHA's constituent health areas could match with the boundaries of the reorganised local authorities.[11]

The chairman and members of each RHA are appointed by the Secretary of State after consultation with the major health professions, main local authorities, universities and relevant trade unions and voluntary bodies. The functions of the RHAs include the activities of the former RHBs, such as manpower planning, major computer and operational research services and the selection, design and construction-management of major capital projects. The new RHAs were required to undertake an enlarged role of service planning, liaison, co-ordination and monitoring for their regions — in line with the reorganisation's objectives of integrating primary, hospital and community care services as fully as possible. Since reorganisation, the evolution of policy on the equalising of health care resources across health regions, areas and districts (see more detailed discussion of this topic in Chapter 8) has further increased the role of RHAs, in respect of planning and administering resource allocation arrangements for their regions, and overseeing and monitoring revenue and capital funding, especially major capital-expenditure programmes.[12] Additionally, the RHAs decide the development of medical specialties and act as the employing authority for consultants and senior registrars of non-teaching AHAs; and also they provide the blood transfusion service, the ambulance service in metropolitan countries and an expanded programme of management services and training.

Each RHA is a corporate body of unpaid members who meet at intervals under a part-time salaried chairman. The RHA is a statutory body corporate, and so its functions are a collective responsibility (to the Secretary of State and the DHSS) of the Authority membership as a whole.[13] The Grey Book specified the functions and role for the RHA as follows:

The line of accountability will run between the statutory Authorities, i.e. AHA to RHA. The RHAs will act as a link between the Secretary

of State and the DHSS. The RHA will be responsible for establishing priorities between the competing claims of AHAs and allocating resources to them in accordance with national guidance on policy. . . . It will also review, challenge and approve AHA plans, and subsequently control AHA performance in relation to agreed plans.[14]
The RHA has to delegate major executive responsibilities to its AHAs and to its Regional officers (for Regionally-developed services), and focus the limited time of its Members on the important issues of policy, planning and resource allocation. The Authority can, therefore, be expected to review proposals on policies and priorities submitted to it by AHAs and by the RTO and decide on Regional policies and priorities within the framework of national policy. The Authority will establish planning guidelines for AHAs on priorities and available resources. Subsequently, it will review objectives, plans and budgets submitted to it annually by AHAs and by the RTO (for Regional services).[15]
In addition the RHA must control the performance of its AHAs and its Regional officers.[16]
A further important responsibility of the RHA will be to assist the Secretary of State to establish realistic national policies and priorities.[17]

It may appear from the above quotations from the Grey Book that a weighty, if not onerous, burden of responsibility hangs upon the shoulders of the members of each RHA. The Grey Book recognises this — in some degree, at least — by stating:

If the RHA is to delegate major responsibilities to AHAs while maintaining ultimate control of AHA performance, it must have strong advice and support from its Regional staff. The Regional Team of Officers (RTO) will therefore be responsible for recommending Regional policies to the RHA and advising on its approval of AHA policies.[18]

The RTO that provides the full-time managerial supervision of the RHA's responsibilities is composed of the following five officers: the Regional Medical Officer and the Regional Nursing Officer (each concerned with the planning of services for their specialisms); the Regional Works Officer (managing staff concerned with the design and construction of major capital developments); the Regional Treasurer (responsible for all financial and accounting services, and for the administration of cash limits and other expenditure controls); and the Regional Administrator (responsible, first, for normal administrative services such as general personnel matters, public relations, and supplies and management services; secondly, for regional-based services such as blood transfusion, ambulance services and central computing services; and thirdly, for providing general co-ordination to the administrative work of the RHA, inclusive of ensuring, e.g. that planning activities and timetables are fulfilled, and that required reports and other information are supplied to the DHSS).[19] In general, all members of the RTO have responsibilities for personnel, education and training matters affecting their own functional specialisms; and also, they all have important involvement with capital-development planning and projects. It is, after all, the most distinctive feature of the RHA's function, that it operates to plan and shape the future scale, location and balance of health services (especially hospital services) through its powers to channel and administer capital expenditure.

Each member of the RTO is individually accountable for his own specialism of activities to both the RTO and the RHA. In addition, the RTO as a group have a collective accountability to the RHA for the discharge of regional responsibilities and for the work of the RTO as a management team.[20] This combination of individual plus collective officer-responsibility is a distinctive feature of the NHS organisation, and it occurs not just at RTO level, but also at the levels of the Area Team of Officers and the District Management Team. This organisational arrangement is interdependent with the concept of 'consensus management', a somewhat controversial approach to managerial co-ordination which will be discussed in more detail in Chapter 12.

Planning is intended to be a key function of each RHA. Planning systems and problems are discussed in Chapters 5 and 9, but here we should at least note the organisational arrangements to assist the RTO and the RHA in their planning functions. The RHA will have service planning teams — with medical, nursing and other professional and technical membership — to study and co-ordinate health care services on a regional, strategic basis. Multidisciplinary teams are set up additionally for each major capital project for which a service planning team has established a need, and a priority has been approved by the RHA. Regional planning is further influenced by the counsel provided by medical and other professional advisory committees that on a representative basis draw upon the experience and viewpoints of medical and other professional staffs working at area and district levels. Such advisory committees can have an important influence not only on long-term planning in a general sense, but also on specific capital developments and on more immediate resource allocation decisions such as the acquisition and allocation of major items of medical and scientific equipment. RHAs have a role of potentially great influence on financial resource allocation more generally, through their authority to interpret and apply RAWP allocations of capital to obtain a balance of resources within each region.

Area Health Authorities

AHAs comprise the lowest level of statutory authority within the health service. Their number (90 in England) and their boundaries were determined by a desire to match AHAs with corresponding metropolitan districts, non-metropolitan counties and, in London, combinations of one to three boroughs — in the hope that through such matching (termed 'coterminosity') more effective joint NHS and local authority planning and co-ordination of community health and personal social services could be achieved. AHAs vary in population from under a quarter-million to over a million.

The chairman of each AHA is appointed by the Secretary of State. However, a majority of AHA members (typically 14 at the time of reorganisation) are appointed by the relevant RHA, with the minority appointed by local authorities and by the university(ies) associated with medical education and research within the region. However, all members of AHAs, as indeed of RHAs, are expected, once appointed, to act in the best interests of the health service and the population served within their authority: that is, the chairman and members serve the AHA in their individual capacities rather than as 'representatives' or 'delegates'.[21]

The Grey Book explains that the AHA should delegate executive responsibilities to its Area Team of Officers (ATO), whilst concentrating its own time on policy, planning and resource allocation decisions, setting area priorities within the framework of national and regional policy.[22] The AHA must review and monitor objectives, plans and budgets prepared by its area and district teams, and it must ensure that its services are planned and co-ordinated alongside those of the local authority.[23] Additionally, the AHA must appoint its principal officers, consult with its professional advisory committees, liaise with the relevant Community Health Councils, establish and liaise with its Family Practitioner Committee, and generally ensure the proper control and reporting of the affairs of the authority and its officers.[24] 'The AHA will itself take all the decisions on policy, planning and resource allocation, and control the performance of its officers.'[25]

Each AHA is supported *both* by its ATO and by the management teams in its constituent health districts. Except for a restricted range of services provided at area level, it is the district-level management teams that actually manage the main resources used to deliver health care to patients at the operational level, especially as regards the hospital services: the functions of these teams will be described in the next section below. The key functions of the ATO consist of advising and supporting the AHA generally; reviewing the plans, resource needs and budgets of health districts in the light of AHA policy and planning guidelines; liaising with local authorities in respect of joint planning and the work of the joint consultative committees; monitoring and reporting on district performance (against plans and budgets, etc.); and managing and being accountable for certain area services.[26] These area-managed services consist of activities thought to be best managed at area level because of the need for co-ordination with equivalent local authorities (e.g. child health, health education, school health and doctors in public health); the need for co-ordination with Family Practitioner Committee services (e.g. dentistry and pharmaceuticals); or the economy or efficiency of more central organisation (e.g. ambulance, supplies and works services and the administration of certain medical, financial and personnel records, etc.).

The ATO consists of four officers. These are the Area Medical Officer, Area Nursing Officer, Area Treasurer and Area Administrator. Whilst not members of the ATO *per se*, there are also other area officers of senior status with the right to attend ATO meetings for discussions affecting their own services: these normally include the Area Dental Officer, Area Pharmaceutical Officer and Area Works Officer. Each member of the ATO has a principal responsibility as a member of the team to join in advising and supporting the AHA. Each has a major responsibility for advising and monitoring the performance of his own function as carried out at district level. In general, each has also to take responsibility for planning and for functional management in his own specialism insofar as it is carried out or administered at area level. For example, the Area Medical Officer has particular responsibility for developing health education programmes, health care information systems, the promotion of research, medical planning and area medical advisory liaison. The Area Administrator has to oversee the work of specialist officers in charge of family practitioner administration, ambulance services, supplies, personnel, management services and capital development – in addition to staff servicing the planning and other information needs of the AHA. The Area Works Officer is concerned with the development and administration of the smaller building projects not administered by the RHA (e.g. health centres), as well as with the co-ordination of area engineering and property maintenance.[27]

Health Districts

The Health District is the operational-level 'building block' of health care management. It is the lowest level of the NHS at which the attempt is made formally to co-ordinate closely the primary, hospital and community care services. Indeed, the notion of the Health District is to a considerable degree born of the desire to integrate the tripartite health services and to reduce the dominance of acute (hospital) care. Nevertheless, the dominant factors governing the size and boundaries of Health Districts, typically, are the criteria of optimal size and catchment area for an efficient (district) general hospital. It was deemed that 200,000 to 250,000 was the optimal population base to relate to a district general hospital, but in the event problems associated with historical catchment areas, variable population densities, pre-existing non-optimal-sized general hospitals, etc., resulted in Health Districts at the time of reorganisation varying between 85,000 and about 500,000 in population.[28]

Health Districts do not have a statutory identity of their own. They are managerial units within their respective AHAs. However, 34 of the 222 Health Districts designated in England and Wales at the time of reorganisation were the sole districts in their respective areas, and have shared the same senior officers for the conduct of both area and district functions (see section on single-district areas below).

Each District Management Team (DMT) was intended to be responsible for effecting planning, integration and co-ordination of the total range of health services.[29] To this end, DMT membership includes two elected (part-time) medical representatives (one a consultant and the other a general practitioner) in addition to four full-time officers whose functions largely mirror their counterparts on the ATO. These officers are the District Community Physician, the District Nursing Officer, the District Finance Officer and the District Administrator. Certain other officers have the right to attend team meetings for the discussion of matters concerning their own services, and moreover if the district is part of a teaching area (AHA(T)), then the dean or other representative of the local university medical school may attend for business concerning the needs of clinical teaching and research.[30] It must be stressed that the DMT does not have the full range of powers over the delivery of health care that, e.g., a company board of directors enjoys over its firm's delivery of manufacturing and sales activities. The actual management of the resources available at the point of contact with patients is largely controlled by the individual consultants and general practitioners, although nurses and paramedical professions are playing a managerial role of growing importance in the application of their own special skills and resources to patient care.

The DMT is intended to be 'a group of equals, no member being the managerial supervisor of another'.[31] In the relevant passages of the Grey Book particular emphasis appears to be laid upon the equality of team members at this, the district level, as also upon the need for the consensus resolution of issues, so that no decisions can be taken that override the opposition of any team member. Presumably this especial emphasis at the level of the DMT is not unrelated to the membership of a consultant and general practitioner: that is, it probably was felt necessary to guarantee that the medical-representative members could not be overruled on a matter they considered to adversely affect the clinical autonomy of the medical professions. The problems that clinical autonomy imposes on national health care management will be considered further in later chapters.

Whilst the DMT is expected to operate by co-operation, consensus and a sense of joint responsibility, it is not to be held 'corporately responsible' in the sense applied to AHAs and RHAs. If the performance of a DMT is considered unacceptable by its AHA, then the AHA, assisted by the area officers, is expected to assess the performance of each member of the DMT to establish the source of difficulty. Each officer of the ATO has the duty on behalf of the AHA to monitor the work of his counterpart on the DMT, even though he does not hold a line-management role of authority over the counterpart.

Amongst the important duties specified for DMTs are the establishment and co-ordination of District Planning Teams (originally described as Health Care Planning Teams) with an integrated (i.e. cross-service) approach to the study and planning of services for particular care groups (e.g. the elderly, mentally handicapped, etc.); the integration of the work and planning of the various skill groups in medical care, irrespective of whether these skills are located in primary, hospital or community care services; and the co-ordination of all health care activities below the district management level.[32]

Turning to the functions of the individual members of the DMT, one must first note the distinctive difference of the DMT, compared to the ATO and the RTO, in respect of the medical representation on the DMT. These representatives (not delegates) are drawn from the District Medical Committee (DMC), and were recommended normally to be the chairman and vice-chairman of the DMC. The DMC itself is intended to be representative of all general practitioners and specialist hospital medical staff in the district, and to co-ordinate medical health care throughout the district.[33] The place of the DMC within the larger framework of overall medical advisory and executive committee structures will be considered separately below.

Turning to the full-time officers on the DMT, the District Community Physician has as his principal responsibilities, first, the co-ordination of preventive (e.g. immunisation) and public health services generally within the district; and secondly, co-ordination of the medical aspects of planning and developing all operational health care services in the district. He should normally obtain assistance from specialists in community medicine attached to the Area Medical Officer's staff, and from support staff (e.g. for health statistics and studies, and for the servicing of District (Health Care) Planning Teams and other committee and local-authority liaison commitments) attached to him by the District Administrator.[34] Indeed the District Community Physician has only very limited staff and technical resources under his own direct and full control, and this has been criticised as weakening his ability to achieve the most effective planning and health care co-ordination. Moreover, many posts for specialists in community medicine are vacant in AHAs, because of a shortage of trained staff.

The District Nursing Officer, like the other officers, has an important role in planning service development. Unlike the District Community Physician (and the two medical representatives on the DMT), the DNO also has a general managerial responsibility for the organisation, manning and performance of the services provided by the nursing profession within the district.[35]

The duties of the District Finance Officer are not dissimilar from those of the Area Treasurer, although the emphasis is relatively less on financial planning and resource allocation, and relatively more on operational budgeting and the detailed control of expenditure.[36]

The District Administrator, like the Area and Regional Administrators, may be described unofficially as having a generalised responsibility for every district activity that is not (i) explicitly the province of another officer, or (ii) a matter of clinical or medical-practitioner professional judgement. He must provide general administrative co-ordination for the DMT and its district staff, oversee the management of administrative services, and be responsible for the management of institutional and support services. Thus he is responsible for personnel and management services, and for co-ordinating the fulfilment of the planning process and timetable. The institutional and support services for which he is responsible include the district catering, cleaning, portering, laundry, transport and property-maintenance services. He is also responsible for the administration of institutions and the co-ordination of services below district level, and for non-professional administrative aspects of the work of the district building and engineering officers, the district pharmaceutical officer and certain paramedical services.[37] The foregoing describes a general model: at district level and below there is a degree of organisational flexibility allowed, so as to adapt to differing local characteristics (e.g. differences in the geographical size and populations of districts, and in the distribution and character of their hospitals and other facilities).

Below District Level

A Health District, on average, covers perhaps a third of a county, but often it is larger. It will include one or more major hospitals, often a number of smaller outlying, community or specialist hospitals, and also a variety of domiciliary and support-service establishments, not to mention health centres and clinics. Especially in the more populous and dispersed districts, it follows that the administration and co-ordination of health services on a local basis may require a level of management between the district level and the level of the individual institution. This applies especially in nursing, the administrative function and such 'hotel' functions as catering. This intermediate level is termed the 'sector' level. The DMT is the lowest level required to act jointly, by consensus. At sector and institution levels management is primarily skill-group centred – i.e. based on the functional-management approach. However, the Grey Book did encourage liaison between skill groups at sub-district levels, and it specified that 'sector administrators' should be responsible for 'managing or coordinating the institutional and support services' within large institutions or sector groupings of institutions.[38]

Single-District Areas

The 34 Health Districts that were created as the sole districts within their areas constitute a special case in respect of organisational arrangements. In this case 'the functions described for the DMT and the ATO will be carried out by an Area Management Team (AMT), which, like a DMT, will include representative clinicians'.[39] In effect, all the activities of an ATO and DMT are conflated into one body, the AMT. The three principal differences from the multi-district area (MDA) appear to be (i) that a clinical view on management issues is more fully represented in the single-district area (SDA) than in the MDA, (ii) that there may be considerable saving of duplication of labour in combining district and area planning and monitoring activities in one single tier of management, and (iii) that AMT members may feel themselves under considerable pressure and tension in simultaneously filling the roles of dispassionate planners of change and advisers to the AHA, whilst carrying functional responsibility for the provision of ongoing services within the district management structure. This and related issues will be considered further in Chapter 12.

Teaching Hospitals

On reorganisation, the undergraduate teaching hospitals were brought under RHAs. They are administered by Teaching Districts under the statutory responsibility of a Teaching Area (Area Health Authority (Teaching) – AHA(T)). The membership of the AHA(T) includes two members nominated by the university (an ordinary AHA has only one) and at least a further two additional members with teaching hospital experience. Postgraduate teaching hospitals (apart from Hammersmith and Northwick Park) are now to remain separate from the regional administration of services. They were assured of independence from the NHS only until February 1979 under the National Health Service Reorganisation Act. However, recently the Secretary of State announced that they would continue to enjoy independent status and be administered by Boards of Governors responsible directly to the Secretary of State.

Family Practitioner Committees

The family practitioner services include medical and dental practitioners, pharmacists and ophthalmic and dispensing opticians. They consist of the primary care professions, who do not work as salaried NHS staff, but who provide NHS services under contractual arrangements on the basis of payment for service rendered. Prior to the NHSS reorganisation, the family practitioner services were organised and administered (as to contracts and finances, etc.) through Executive Councils largely matched with local authorities to assist liaison on matters of joint interest to the primary care and community care services. The Executive Councils were funded directly from the DHSS. At reorganisation, the Executive Councils were replaced by Family

Practitioner Committees (FPCs) based upon the reorganised local authority and AHA boundaries. Direct funding from the DHSS was retained, but for purposes of general liaison and reporting the new FPCs were made accountable corporately to the new AHAs. Typically, each FPC has 30 members, eleven nominated by the AHA, four by local authorities and the other 15 by the local medical committee and other professional committees. The FPC inherited duties concerned with the provision and location of family practitioner services, and the publishing of lists thereof; contract management and validation, and payment of practitioner fees and costs; and certain complaints procedures. At reorganisation, the FPC was made a statutory committee of the AHA, and the FPC Finance Officer and Administrator were made accountable to their ATO counterparts in respect of the technical performance of their work, and for the FPC's work on health centre and attachment schemes. There is normally some membership in common between the FPC and the AHA, and this, plus the organisational changes above, was intended to encourage a greater degree of co-ordination of primary care with hospital and community care services.[40] The direct and separate financing of the FPC was no doubt retained in order to reassure the FPC practitioners that their independent contractual status was not threatened. Nevertheless, there is also a difference in kind between FPC expenditure and the other expenditure of AHAs and RHAs. FPC expenditure is open-ended, in the sense that the DHSS is obliged to reimburse all the fees and costs incurred under practitioner contracts. These fees and costs depend partly on patient morbidity and demand, and partly on the manner in which practitioners respond to patient demands and needs. In particular, the cost of drugs and other prescriptions constitutes a major element of cost that is not currently controlled by budgets or cash limits.

Medical (Advisory) Committees

There are statutory advisory committees at area and regional levels: the Regional Medical Advisory Committee (RMAC) and the Area Medical Advisory Committee (AMAC). The Grey Book, however, focused on clinical involvement at district level. We discuss problems of involving clinicians in planning arising from this emphasis in Chapters 5 and 9. Here we indicate the potential for duplication and confusion in the provision of clinical advice.

At each level the Medical Committee includes the community physician, hospital-based doctors and general practitioners. The District Medical Committee is not intended to deal with the organisation of medical work in hospitals or general practice, but rather to provide a common forum for matters of policy which involve both. General practitioners have their own local Medical Committee. Hospital-based doctors could be organised by specialty through the Cogwheel structure and/or by hospital through a Hospital Medical Staff Committee. Clinicians may also be involved in planning teams at district level (Health Care Planning Teams/District Planning Teams) and have representatives on DMTs. In a MDA members of the AMAC may be uncertain as to whether they are to represent their specialty or their district. Moreover, many individual clinicians are uncertain of the appropriate forum, from the many available, for the resolution of clinical matters.

Joint Consultative Committees

During the years of study and debate that culminated in the reorganisation of the NHS, it was often argued that the key justification for reorganisation was the need to integrate the established NHS functions of primary and hospital health care more closely with the community health care and other personal social services administered by local authorities. In Northern Ireland health and personal social services were brought together formally under reorganised Health Boards.[41] In Great Britain the reorganisation transferred community and school health to the NHS, but left the main personal social services to be administered by the local authorities. Personal social services that relate to the welfare of children, the elderly and the handicapped, are examples of services that impinge on the NHS – and vice versa. For example, elderly people requiring intermittent medical supervision in many cases could be accommodated either in NHS institutions or in local-community domiciliary accommodation.

Whilst on a day-to-day basis there should be frequent contacts and acts of co-operation between NHS staff and social services staff, it was considered desirable after the 1974 reorganisation to create a formal vehicle for consultation and for the development of joint interests between each AHA and its local authorities. The vehicle is the Joint Consultative Committee (JCC), which is assisted between meetings by working parties of senior officers from both types of authority.[42]

The period of reorganisation coincided with a period of economic difficulty for the nation, when the growth rate of both health and local authority funding was reduced. This was frustrating to JCC activity and progress, as often the developments that occupied the grey area of divided or shared responsibility between the two kinds of authorities (e.g. residential accommodation for the mentally ill and handicapped, and day centres and domiciliary assistance for the elderly) would appear to each authority to be a reasonable area for its own retrenchment in the growth of spending. To counter this situation the DHSS announced earmarked capital funding that would be used for the construction of JCC-approved capital projects, with a view to their subsequent management by local authorities from their revenue funds. Whilst spending of no more than £50m annually may be involved, this capital injection appears to have given some hope that JCCs may indeed contribute usefully to the improved community care of relevant client groups, and to the integration or at least co-ordination of relevant health and social services planning at the local level.[43]

Community Health Councils

Whereas JCCs match AHAs to provide a meeting ground for professional staff from both local authorities and health areas and districts to work together on (primarily) community care co-ordination and development, Community Health Councils (CHCs) provide a forum, at the level of the Health District, for the expression of the views of local users of the health services. The 1974 reorganisation transferred community health from local authority to NHS control, and thus terminated the local authority health committees through which local and user views on health care had been available. The reorganisation also terminated the old hospital management committees, so that these two changes together had the effects of reducing the number of contacts between local, lay opinion and the NHS, and of removing such contact to the more remote level of the AHA. The CHCs were conceived partly as a counterweight to the above changes, and partly as a positive move towards reflecting the views of health service users *per se* – as distinct from local authority spokesmen for such users. As a result of further considerations such as were argued in *Democracy in the NHS*[44] the role of the CHCs was further strengthened in 1975.[45]

CHCs have between 18 and 36 members, depending on the size of the Health District. Half the members are nominated by the local authorities, one-third by voluntary bodies and the remainder by the RHA. The RHA formally appoints the members, for four-year terms with half of the membership being renewed every two years. Most CHCs subdivide into working groups matched to particular sectors of health care, and they conduct investigations, make visits, consider information and prepare reports – although in the sector of family practitioner services their formal powers of enquiry are more restricted than elsewhere. The formal meetings of the CHCs are open to public attendance (as also are AHA and RHA meetings). One member of the CHC may attend and speak at AHA meetings, but not vote. There is a statutory annual public meeting jointly held between the CHC and the AHA. Also the CHC must be consulted on certain matters, most notably all proposals for hospital closures. Each CHC must submit an annual report to its RHA.[46]

CHCs have been a controversial innovation in some districts, first on the general ground of their meddling and using up resources (i.e. the cost of their administration and expenses, and the time of medical and administrative staff taken up in servicing their information requirements) that could be better spent on actual health care; and secondly on the more specific ground of some CHCs allegedly having been irresponsibly obstructive in certain cases of proposed hospital closure. As regards the first and more general argument, it seems obvious that health care is a field where the individual consumer at his time of need has little opportunity to influence the standards of care and compassion that he receives, so that some collective machinery for voicing consumer needs and values is justifiable: it is not obvious that this could be achieved in any better way than through the CHCs. Regarding the second point, it is a matter for personal judgement whether or not some CHCs have been unreasonably obstructive over hospital closures. What may be of greater long-term importance is the possibility that some CHCs have been influenced by local-authority political point-scoring, and/or by worker-group pressures for job preservation. Local authorities, whether viewed as administrative entities or as entities of local political will, have other channels for influencing the local health services. Similarly, the trade unions have their proper and agreed channels for influence and grievance. The CHCs should focus their concern strictly on the needs and best interests of health service *consumers*.

The Health Service Commissioner

The role of the Health Service Commissioner (which extends to England, Wales and Scotland) is to investigate complaints from individual members of the public, as well as to deal with enquiries and requests for advice. Members of the public have direct access to the Commissioner's office, provided only that they shall have first made their complaints to the Health Authority concerned, and allowed reasonable time for a response. In 1977–8 a total of 584 complaints were received. 364 complaints were rejected, of which 33 per cent because they involved clinical judgement, 19 per cent because

Authorities had not been given a chance to answer, and the balance for various reasons of falling outside the Commissioner's authority.[47] During 1977–78 109 complaint investigations were completed and reports issued, and varying degrees of justification for complaint were found in 67 cases. The most frequent causes of some justification in complaint were failure to supply information to patients or relatives, unhelpful attitudes, failings in day-to-day administration and the handling of complaints by Authorities. The role of the Commissioner does not appear to have a major impact on the NHS, although generally seen as a desirable and non-controversial safeguard of the public interest. There is controversy, however, as regards the possibility of extending the Commissioner's jurisdiction to include complaints involving clinical judgement, as was recommended in a Select Committee report published late in 1977.[48]

Organisational Differences in Wales, Scotland and Northern Ireland

The Absence of a Regional Tier

An important difference between England and the other countries of the UK is that there are regional authorities in England only. In each of the other countries its Health Department fulfils a mixture of the functions of the English DHSS and an English RHA, although for some functions the responsibilities of the latter may be devolved to (Area) Health Authorities – or there is even the risk that they may not be fully discharged.[49] Staff both in the Health Departments and in Health Authorities valued the close and direct links between area and governmental levels. In Wales, for instance, there are regular meetings between the Secretary of State and the chairmen of the AHAs, and between the different team members (administrators, treasurers, nursing officers, medical officers) and their civil service counterparts.

The Composition of Teams of Officers at Area Level

In Scotland, Boards are served by an Area Executive Group (AEG) of four officers, whether they be Single or Multi-District Boards. These teams are directly analogous to the four officers who comprise the ATO in Multi-District Areas in England and Wales:

Scotland (AEG)	*England and Wales (ATO)*
Chief Administrative Medical Officer	Area Medical Officer
Chief Area Nursing Officer	Area Nursing Officer
Treasurer	Area Treasurer
Secretary	Area Administrator

In Northern Ireland the Area Executive Committee Team has five members:

Chief Administrative Officer
Chief Administrative Medical Officer
Chief Administrative Nursing Officer
Director of Social Services
Chairman of the Medical Advisory Committee

The three significant differences of this team from those of England, Scotland and Wales are: the inclusion of the Director of Social Services and the Chairman of the Medical Advisory Committee, and the omission of the Finance Officer.

The Membership and Structure of Area Health Authorities and Boards

Members in Wales, Scotland and Northern Ireland are generally appointed by the Secretary of State. In Wales, four of the 15 members are appointed by the matching county council. In Scotland the Secretary of State appoints members nominated by health care professions, trade unions, universities and other organisations. A similar practice is followed in Northern Ireland.

In England, AHAs, according to the Grey Book, are not supposed to have standing committees.[50] In Scotland the Health Board we visited had formed a planning committee – although this consisted of all its members. In Northern Ireland, Boards are served by four committees: Policy and Resources, Social Services, Health Services and Administrative Services.

District/Area Relationships

In England there is no line relationship between members of DMTs and ATOs nor is there a line relationship between these teams. The general principle for the management by areas of districts is that the former should exercise a monitoring and co-ordinating role with respect to the latter. The AHA is expected to resolve differences between areas and districts, and the part-time chairman is the person to whom members of district and area teams are directly accountable (in an area with three districts this means that sixteen professional staff report to him). In Scotland, Wales and Northern Ireland, there is a line relationship between officers at area and district level. In England, the Kogan Report found a greater element of tension and dissatisfaction in area/district relationships than in region/area relationships; with 'a greater wish for control by the Area officers, and for autonomy by the district officers'.[51] But the area/district relationships in the rest of the UK were often seen to be more strained and tense than in England and the complaints put more sharply.[52]

The District Organisation

In England and Wales two clinicians are included on DMTs. These are elected by the District Medical Committee. In Northern Ireland the chairman of the District Medical Advisory Committee is a member of the District Executive Team. In Scotland there is no clinician as member of the District Executive Group. The District teams of the four countries are:

England and Wales	*Northern Ireland*	*Scotland*
District Nursing Officer	District Administrative Nursing Officer	District Nursing Officer
District Administrator	District Administrative Officer	District Administrator
District Community Physician	District Administrative Medical Officer	District Medical Officer
District Finance Officer		District Finance Officer
Consultant Representative		
GP Representative	Chairman of the District Medical Advisory Committee	
	District Social Services Officer	

Involvement of Clinicians

Clinicians are involved directly on DMTs in England, Wales and Northern Ireland. In England and Wales clinicians are not members of ATOs in Multi-District Areas, but in Northern Ireland the Chairman of the AMC is a member of the AET. In Scotland the view was taken that it would be better if the Medical Advisory Committees were not directly involved in the reorganised administrative structure: the position of all chairmen of Medical Advisory Committees was believed to be strengthened by their independence. However, the Scottish Home and Health Department (SHHD) has recently undertaken a review of the medical advisory structure with a view to reform its shortcomings.[53]

Medical Advisory Committees exist at regional, area and district levels in England, and at country, area and district levels in the other countries of the UK. In Scotland, advice to the SHHD is channelled through the National Medical Consultative Committee, in Wales there is a Welsh Medical Advisory Committee similarly organised as Regional Medical Advisory Committees in England; and in Northern Ireland there is a central Medical Advisory Committee.

Community Health Councils and Local Health Councils

In England and Wales half the members of the CHC are appointed by the local authorities. In England the RHA, and in Wales the Welsh Office, is responsible for appointing the nominees for the other positions, funding the operating expenses and providing training opportunities. In Scotland and Northern Ireland the CHC equivalents are called Local Health Councils and District Committees, respectively. Health Boards are responsible for establishing these bodies in each country and each reports to its respective Board.

Conclusion

In this chapter we have summarised the organisation of the NHS as factually and dispassionately as we could manage. Clearly the 1974 reorganisation, together with concurrent developments, brought relatively sudden and drastic change to the working relationships of NHS managers and other professional staff, as to the direct influence that individual clinicians could exert upon the local management process. All this, plus a rise in the share of administrative costs within the total costs of the NHS inevitably provoked complaint and controversy concerning the wisdom, effectiveness and value for money of the reorganisation. We examine many of the specific issues of controversy in later chapters of this book, and in particular we examine issues of organisational management structure in Chapter 12.

Notes

1. Ruth Levitt, *The Reorganised National Health Service,* 2nd edn (Croom Helm, London, 1977). Although this excellent book concentrates upon the post-1974 reorganised NHS, it also includes a concise history of the NHS and its organisation up to 1974. We are indebted to this book for information and insights reflected in this and other chapters.

2. *The National Health Service Reorganisation Act, 1973* (HMSO, London, 1973).

3. Department of Health and Social Security (DHSS), *Management Arrangements for the Reorganised National Health Service* (the Grey Book) (HMSO,

London, 1972).
   4. Ibid., para. 2.33.
   5. Ibid.
   6. Ibid., para. 2.34.
   7. Ibid.
   8. Ibid.
   9. Ibid.
  10. Levitt, *Reorganised NHS*, pp. 28-39.
  11. Ibid., pp. 39-43.
  12. DHSS, *Sharing Resources for Health in England*, Report of the Resource Allocation Working Party (the RAWP Report) (HMSO, London, 1976).
  13. Grey Book, para. 2.26.
  14. Ibid., para. 2.24.
  15. Ibid., para. 2.27.
  16. Ibid., para. 2.28.
  17. Ibid., para. 2.29.
  18. Ibid., para. 2.30.
  19. Ibid., pp. 39-44.
  20. Ibid., para. 2.32.
  21. Levitt, *Reorganised NHS*, Ch. 3 for discussion of AHAs.
  22. Grey Book, para. 2.8.
  23. Ibid.
  24. Ibid., paras. 2.9–2.11.
  25. Ibid., para. 2.11.
  26. Ibid., paras. 2.18–2.22.
  27. Ibid., paras. 2.74–2.81.
  28. Levitt, *Reorganised NHS*, pp. 68–9.
  29. Grey Book, paras. 2.39–2.40.
  30. Ibid., paras. 2.41–2.42.
  31. Ibid., para. 2.42.
  32. Ibid., para. 2.39 ff.
  33. Ibid., para. 2.55.
  34. Ibid., paras. 2.57–2.58.
  35. Ibid., paras. 2.59–2.60.
  36. Ibid., paras. 2.61–2.62.
  37. Ibid., paras. 2.63–2.65.
  38. Ibid., paras. 2.67–2.68.
  39. Ibid., para. 2.23.
  40. Levitt, *Reorganised NHS*, p. 66.
  41. *The Working of the National Health Service*, Royal Commission on the NHS, Research Paper No. 1 (HMSO, London, 1978), pp. 51–5. *Management of Financial Resources in the National Health Service*, Royal Commission on the NHS, Research Paper No. 2 (HMSO, London, 1978), p. 231 ff.
  42. Levitt, *Reorganised NHS*, pp. 62–3.
  43. Ibid., pp. 86–7.
  44. DHSS, *Democracy in the National Health Service* (HMSO, London, 1974).
  45. Levitt, *Reorganised NHS*, pp. 191–5.
  46. Ibid.
  47. Health Service Commissioner, *Annual Report for 1977–78* (HMSO, London, 1978).
  48. Select Committee on the Independent Review of Hospital Complaints in the National Health Service, *First Report of the Select Committee on the Parliamentary Commissioner for Administration; Session 1977–78*, HC45 (December 1977).

49. The Scottish Home and Health Department (SHHD) did not issue guidance on reorganisation in a single document, but through circulars, etc. The Welsh Office and Northern Ireland Office published equivalent documents to the Grey Book: Welsh Office, *The Management Arrangements for the NHS in Wales* (HMSO, Cardiff, 1972); Northern Ireland Office, *An Integrated Service: The Reorganisation of Health and Social Services in Northern Ireland* (February 1972).

50. Grey Book, para. 2.11.

51. *The Working of the National Health Service,* p. 30.

52. Ibid.

53. SHHD, *The Medical Advisory Structure Within Health Boards in Scotland, A Review* (1977).

4 THE PROCESSES OF RESOURCE ALLOCATION

The Economic and Financial Contexts of Public Expenditure Planning and Control

The volume of resources available to the NHS for the medium term (the current year and four forward years) is decided through the Public Expenditure Survey. The cash allocations for the coming year are embodied in the Estimates process. We describe each of these processes in the sections that follow. We begin by describing the economic and financial contexts in which public expenditure is planned and controlled, in order to throw light on why it is so difficult for governments to meet the continued demand for more resources for the NHS – a matter which we explore in Chapter 7.

The Legislative Financial Framework

The Crown (in effect, successive governments) is responsible for financing its expenditure by levying taxes, or by borrowing. It has a wide discretion as to whether it proposes to the House of Commons a balance of expenditure and revenue, or a surplus or a deficit; and it has complete legal freedom in the amount it borrows. (In this it is unlike local authorities in the UK and some foreign governments – e.g. USA, France and Germany – but it is like some foreign municipalities such as the unfortunate New York City.) Before the war a 'balanced budget' was the convention: this was concerned with Government (or 'Exchequer') finances only. (It meant that taxes and other income met 'above-the-line' expenditure – that is, expenditure which was not met directly out of borrowing.) From the Second World War onwards, however, the Government's financial balance (however defined) has been seen, at least in part, as a tool for keeping the desired balance of demand and supply *in the economy as a whole*. This has been technically possible because there are no limits to the Treasury's *borrowing* powers,[1] though there are statutory controls on what it may *lend* (usually in total for a given purpose) and on what it may *spend* for a given purpose in a given year. *Taxation,* however, is specifically authorised by Parliament, some of it on an annual basis, and the Budget is the occasion on which these powers are reviewed, renewed or changed.

Fiscal Management of the Economy

Post-war economic and financial management has used the tool of budgetary (or 'fiscal') management to achieve objectives wider than the economical management of Government finance and the equity of the tax structure. Ministers have had one or more of the following aims: preserving full employment, removing overheating in the economy, or an overseas deficit, encouraging investment and reducing inflation; in part this management has been aimed at countering cyclical movements in the economy, and in part it has had longer-term economic aims. The aim has also been at different times to increase or to decrease the longer-term redistribution of income and wealth, and to improve the incentives to workers, managers and investors.

Thus the tool of budgetary management has been available to ministers for purposes beyond Government finance, though it has not always achieved what was intended. And indeed, the Government is now held responsible for developments throughout the economy — prosperity and growth, unemployment, inflation — even though these result from a multitude of *private* decisions and negotiations. There have been long-term policy declarations about full employment made by governments during and after the war. Thus, the Budget is not just a matter of knowing what taxes and borrowing are going to be needed to cover public spending policies, it is also part of plans for the regulation or encouragement of these various economic developments in accordance with what the electorate now expects of ministers.

This means that policies leading to public expenditure have to be developed in the context of medium-term projections of the economy. But they must also fit in with policies on taxation and on public borrowing. At a given time the critical consideration may be either economic (unemployment or overheating) or financial. Unfortunately, the economic and financial considerations do not always march together. In the last few years it has become clear that the Government cannot in practice continue indefinitely to borrow extremely large sums (over £10,000m Public Sector Borrowing Requirement in 1975–6). After all, someone has to be willing to lend, and in conditions of inflation and lack of confidence in financial management our borrowing may have to be achieved at high and increasing interest rates. This is (in the briefest summary) why limits have been set on borrowing, even though unemployed resources might be put to work if more were spent and borrowed. Because there are also limits on the taxation that can be raised in practice (since increases in taxes can encourage inflationary wage demands or discourage investment and growth), it is not possible to increase the total of public expenditure without limit. That means that many services such as health will not develop as fast as governments and others would like. Decisions like this are only taken after most painful examination and dispute. We examine this subject further in Chapter 7.

The responsibility, within the Cabinet, for the planning and maintenance of this financial and economic balancing act lies with the Chancellor of the Exchequer and (on the expenditure side) the Chief Secretary to the Treasury. They are advised and assisted by Treasury officials, including economists, working in conjunction with the Revenue Departments (on taxation), the Bank of England (on monetary matters) and other ministers and officials concerned with relevant issues such as industry, wages, prices and poverty.

It is a very big task to assemble information which can lead to well-informed judgements by the Chancellor or by the Cabinet. One has to knit together the policies which lead to spending (which means most of the activities of government, central and local) with the prospects for Government finance, for the money supply and the balance of overseas payments, for inflation and for investment and consumption and economic growth. One must then develop policy options which work within all the constraints and which not only help towards the financial and industrial aims of the Government, but also move towards social aims relating to the poverty or prosperity of families and individuals.

This exercise takes place in a kaleidoscope of outside changes, of continued inflation and of uncertainty about what has been happening in the recent past, and how intentions are changing in the private sector. Recommendations have to be made by a certain date so that decisions can be taken, and Parliament and the country can be told in an orderly fashion what is proposed. The decisions are taken by the Cabinet, after examination from the point of view of responsible ministers with many different points of view and responsibilities.

Forecasts and policy changes are made more than once a year. However, there is an annual cycle (including the Public Expenditure Survey) which results in decisions on public expenditure each winter, and on taxation each spring. This is directly linked with the process of allocation and budgeting in the health service, and with the management of other functional expenditure programmes.

The Annual Cycle of the Public Expenditure Survey

Treasury Instructions

In the late autumn the Treasury issues instructions (approved by ministers) to spending departments on the assumptions to be used for the survey. Some of these will be economic assumptions also used in parallel forecasting exercises: the most important point however, is the method of working out each spending programme. This may be (i) to assume a continuation of 'existing policies' (an elastic phrase in skilled hands) or (ii) to work out, within given sums related in some arithmetical way to the present programme, what the department would spend this money on, and what the results are intended to be. In recent years it appears that (i) has been followed, rather than (ii). These survey instructions are only a basis for exposition, not decisions on allocation (which will be taken by ministers about a year later). Another point for decision is whether the programmes should show the results of possible upward and downward variations.

Departmental Submissions

Departments then draw up programmes for which they are responsible for the current and next four financial years. The price basis used is known as 'survey prices'; this is a constant price base for each survey and, in practice, departments use the latest prices paid — not future prices; and programmes have to be revalued each year to the new set of prevailing prices. Negotiations on the survey are based on the prices current at (or before) the survey begins. The programmes are sent to the Treasury by a given date in late February, at official level, although each department may already have had to refer some points to its own ministers to ensure that the programme is, within its arbitrary and perhaps restricted total, in line with the ministerial priorities in that Department.

Bilateral Discussions

Officials for each department then enter into a long examination of each programme with the Treasury Expenditure Division concerned. This is designed not so much to arrive at decisions (though some changes may be made as a result of Treasury challenge) as to give figures and text for a fair assessment of each programme *when set alongside the fourteen other programmes* covered by the survey.

The Preparation of the PESC Report

A draft report, embodying the outcome of this work, is then put by the Treasury to the Public Expenditure Survey Committee (PESC). This consists of the Principal Finance Officers (PFOs) from the spending departments, and of officials from Treasury Expenditure Divisions and from the Central Policy Review Staff and perhaps others, under Treasury chairmanship. The PFOs will have been kept in personal touch with the way the survey has been going, both by their own staff and by the chairman, and they will have been told about economic and financial prospects. It is a vital part of the system that the PFOs (who are departmental, not Treasury, officials) should see not only their own problem and something of that of each spending colleague, but also the central problem. There is a high degree of openness and trust between PFOs and the Treasury (indeed the whole survey would be of little reliability or value without this), and this coexists with the loyalty of each PFO to his own minister. The PESC Report which is prepared under their supervision must isolate those points which cannot be settled by officials, and must give clear and practical guidance to ministers on how the choice of priorities can best be approached. It will *not* recommend what those priorities should be: this is the political decision which ministers have to make when analysis has gone as far as it can go. (It will be clear that the *qualitative* assessments by officials are very important; this underlines the importance of efficient departmental information systems, and output measures where possible, and sensitivity to what happens where the health service (for instance) impinges on patients.)

Presentation of the PESC Report to Cabinet by the Chancellor

The PESC Report is addressed to the Chancellor of the Exchequer, though it is designed for all Cabinet Ministers to consider. The Chancellor has by this time (May/June) had the results of the medium-term economic assessments; he has already presented his Budget and made changes in taxation relating to the next year or so; and he now has to consider, with Treasury advice, how the expenditure plans in the survey fit in with the economic forecasts and the prospects for revenue and for borrowing. He knows that the survey has been conducted on certain arbitrary assumptions (explained above) as to the total of each programme. His first step is to put a paper to the Cabinet (together perhaps with a paper by the Chief Secretary on the survey itself). The Chancellor's paper will describe the economic and financial prospects, and will recommend the totals to which public expenditure should be held in one or more key years. These totals may be above or below the survey figures, but in the all-too-common crisis years they are likely to be below. He will seek to get Cabinet agreement on these *total* figures.

Negotiation on Allocations to Programmes

When a decision is reached on these totals (in the early summer) it is necessary to decide on allocations *between* programmes. An *ad hoc* process of discussion and negotiation takes place over the next few months, with the Chief Secretary in the lead. Ideally in the autumn, but sometimes in practice later, the discussions have got to a point when recommendations can be made to the Cabinet, subject to a quite small number of important points which the Cabinet itself will be asked to settle.

Indications to Local Authorities

By this point in the autumn there have been discussions and negotiations with representatives of local authorities about their prospective policies and expenditure. Revenue expenditure by local authorities is not finally, or indeed effectively, controlled by the Government, but it forms parts of the total of public expenditure which (in everyone's interest) is planned for a few years ahead. Furthermore, Government departments concerned with (e.g.) education, housing and personal social services have an influence, which may be strong, on the policies and standards which local authorities adopt, and hence on the level of expenditure. Before the Rate Support Grant for the following financial year is settled in November, the Government will wish to have given the local authorities an indication of its attitude towards those public expenditure programmes where there is doubt about the degree of expansion or contraction, since the local element in those programmes affects the calculation of the relevant expenditure on which the Government gives the Rate Support Grant. This has to be done in time for local authorities to work out their rates for the coming financial year. For this reason, if for no other, decisions on allocations cannot be delayed indefinitely.

Final Cabinet Decisions on Programme Totals

The Cabinet will meet, perhaps several times in a difficult year, to take decisions on the remaining points of allocation. There may be pressure to increase total expenditure because the decisions are too difficult: this underlines the need for clear understanding and decision at the meeting in the early summer. Eventually decisions are taken in the autumn or winter, and officials get instructions accordingly. There may or may not be an early public announcement about policy changes.

Preparation of the Public Expenditure White Paper

Allocations are sorted out at some stage for Scotland and Wales. (These allocations cut across the programmes, which relate to Great Britain or to the whole United Kingdom.[2]) The PFO and the Treasury Division agree a detailed table for each programme for later publication. The drafting of the White Paper on Public Expenditure then begins: the Treasury will prepare the explanation and decisions relating to total expenditure and the economic and financial background; PFOs and Treasury Divisions agree the text describing for each programme the policies which ministers have decided on, and show the intended results of the expenditure on those policies. The whole White Paper (including substantial statistical material) is then approved by ministers, with amendment as necessary.

Publication of the White Paper

The White Paper is published at some time in the winter.[3] The original idea, ten years ago, was to publish in the autumn so that a newly-constituted House of Commons Select Committee on Expenditure could consider the programmes and have time to report to the House before the estimates of government expenditure (resulting from the policies described in the White Paper) were discussed and 'voted'. The object of the Government and the House was to make parliamentary control of finance more than a rather empty formality. But this has never quite worked, and in the last three years the White Paper has been issued in February, January and January respectively, not long before the estimates are presented. (The individual programmes have, according to a recent practice, been examined by subcommittees of the Select Committee on Expenditure, which report through the committee to the House in the coming months.[4]) But although it is not formally linked to the control by the Commons over expenditure, the White Paper is a very important document: it sets out policies and expenditure side by side in comparable form; it pins to the mast the Government's decision both on totals of expenditure and on the description of present policies and aims, making possible monitoring by the House and others, and it explains why (often unwelcome) decisions on allocations have been necessary. We emphasise that ministers collectively are committed to these decisions, even if they were originally opposed to them.

The Estimates Process

The plans of the Public Expenditure Survey are translated into annual cash allocations by Estimates presented to the House of Commons for each financial year. The House of Commons votes money (called 'supplies') for stated purposes, but only on the recommendation of the Crown – that is, on the initiative of the Government. (This is very different from the US system, where Congress can initiate expenditure and override the intentions of the President.) A formal expenditure proposal by the Government, in an estimate, is normally treated as a matter of confidence in the Government's policies *as a whole*: if the House of Commons overthrows the Government's spending proposals at *any* point, the Government normally falls.

Deriving the Estimates from the Survey

Each spending department presents to the Treasury its estimates for the coming year derived from 'year 2' of the White Paper. (In 1979 there is the first stage of a major change, in that estimates are to be assimilated with cash limits (see below), and expressed at prices forecast for the coming year. But for clarity we will describe the separate processes of estimates and cash limits on the basis that has so far been familiar.) The first step is to revalue the figures to prices ruling a year later (roughly those in the autumn just past). Sums required to be voted for each service for each department (which may only cover part of the United Kingdom) are set out in a form which is different from (but as near as possible to) the programmes in the survey and the White Paper. These are examined by the Treasury; they will contain points of detail not covered in the survey and be more up to date. After approval by the Chief Secretary they are presented to the House of Commons in February and March. (On health they are not very informative because of the large amount of authority delegated to Health Departments, and by them to Health Authorities, but they are the basis of parliamentary control and accounting.)

The Cash Limits System

In the last three years these estimates have been reinforced by governmental (not parliamentary) 'cash limits'. These became necessary because the degree of inflation, and its variability between types of expenditure, made it impossible to control expenditure efficiently by the old method of estimate and supplementary estimate (presented at various times during the year in which money was being spent). The cash limit relates to certain parts of public expenditure only. Expenditure by local authorities is not limited in this way, though the Rate Support Grant in aid of their expenditure is. Certain large items of central government expenditure are excluded, notably the cost of the family practitioner services (including drugs), and expenditure on unemployment and other social security benefits, where the entitlement of each individual is controlled by law, but the total cost depends on the numbers who happen to be eligible. The cash limit is set by revaluing the approved programmes to prices expected by the Treasury to apply in the financial year in question for the types of expenditure involved. This revaluation is done as late as possible, so as to get the best forecast data; it is based on forecasts for fairly broad economic categories of expenditure, and not on the detailed revaluations performed in departments for past periods. In effect the Government has been saying, 'We expect the cash cost of this service to be £x, taking into account the inflation we foresee but not assuming our policies against inflation will fail. Spending departments must keep within this figure, and we will not present supplementary estimates to the House which go beyond those implied in this cash limit. If there are ups and downs in prices compared with our forecast, departments will be able to spend rather less, or more, than is shown in the programmes in the White Paper in volume terms. It is only if prices get thoroughly out of hand that we will listen to requests for more money.' In fact, the cash limits, once set, have for the most part held – an exception being the additional sterling cost of overseas services arising from the fall in the exchange rate in 1976–7.

They have been revised – a real, if delicate, distinction from being broken – following public service pay awards in the spring of 1979 whose amount was not known at the time the original limit had to be set; this occurred just before the change from a Labour to Conservative Government, whose attitude to cash limits has not yet been fully revealed.

The Assimilation of Cash Limits with the Estimates

The change being made as we write is that estimates for 1979–80 have (with the Select Committee's agreement) been based on the same forecast prices as cash limits. Therefore the governmental control over expenditure (with the exceptions already noted) will be reinforced by the House of Commons, since the House will now *not* normally expect to see supplementary estimates for the purpose of dealing with price inflation after the main estimates were presented.

The Effects of Cash Limits

Cash limits relate to departmental payments during the year. For the Health Departments, much of their payments consist of bulk issues of cash (for all purposes) to Health Authorities. It is thus the receipt of cash by Health Authorities that is effectively limited.

Whether under cash limits or not, money voted by the House of Commons for a department is for use in a given financial year. Next year's vote is a separate operation which (in principle) takes account of progress in the first year. Late in the financial year there is some incentive to spend amounts which would otherwise not be drawn from the Government's central finances (the Consolidated Fund). Health Authorities have much the same problem when their expenditure in a given year is limited, whether on a cash basis or not. If a department has spent rather more than it was intended to, it has to cut back its expenditure and its services if no more supplementary estimates are possible. This may happen with the system of cash limits; if, for example, inflation turns out to be greater than allowed for by the cash limit. If a department does overspend, the practice is to cut its cash limit in the following year. Health Authorities, like other large public spenders, find it onerous that their spending in real terms may be reduced below the amount originally planned, if the cash limit set by the Government included too little allowance for inflation. Their difficulties are eased by carry-forward arrangements not available to spending departments generally.

To the extent that cash limits are meant to provide a single final and binding allocation of annual funding to the public services concerned, inclusive of inflation allowances, it follows naturally that in the face of economic uncertainties the Government will seek to delay as long as feasible before announcing the cash limits, so as to take account of the latest forecasts of inflation rates. This can mean that Health Authorities may have to start operations in a given budget year without final knowledge of their cash limits. Regional Health Authorities will have been told their allocations in volume terms some months before the start of the financial year. Subregional allocations ought to have been agreed to provide a basis for setting provisional budgets (even if cash allocations are not known), and for translating volume allocations and provisional budgets into cash when cash limits are announced. This translation should not be too difficult because some 75 per cent of all Health Authority spending is on wages, salaries and fees for which the rates for the coming year will have been agreed previously, so that the uncertainty factor in the cash-limits award relates only to the 25 per cent or so of spending on bought-in goods and services. But whilst the Government's cash limit is based upon projections of the '45 Sample Hospital Formula' and other relevant information, individual Health Authorities and Districts will not necessarily view the final allocation and budget-setting process as a simple scaling exercise, especially since in many authorities the critical part of budgeting concerns 'growth money' (see below). Rather, they will have their own opinions on how 'tight' or 'loose' the cash limit looks. Given the recent slowdown in NHS growth, the growth money built in to the real-volume funding forecasts used in the first shot by the DHSS at agreeing target allocations and budgets may often be less than one per cent of total funds. Therefore, if the cash limits when announced appear to contain any possibility of, say, one per cent slack – or the opposite – it follows that at the margin local priorities may dictate some detailed adjustment between separate allocations and budgets.

Reaching the necessary agreements for final cash allocations to budget holders can take a number of weeks after regional cash limits have been announced by the DHSS: difficult and delicate negotiations have still to take place and several tiers are involved.

Carry-forward and Virement

A second constraint on Health Authorities is that capital and revenue are allocated separately, as part of central control over the pace of development, and to avoid embarrassment in management of the economy. RHAs have in fact been given two concessions which allow end-of-year financial flexibility. First, in recent years they have been allowed to carry forward (i.e. defer) spending up to one per cent of their revenue allocations until the next year, and up to ten per cent of their capital allocations until the next year but one. Additionally, they have been allowed to 'vire' (i.e. convert) up to one per cent of revenue allocation into capital funds during the year, or up to ten per cent of capital funds into revenue spending. These facilities help in the practical management problems when inflation rates differ from the rates allowed for in the cash limits, and when technical and labour problems and the weather affect the timing of new developments.

Allocations to Health Departments

In the United Kingdom there are four Health Departments – the Department of Health and Social Security, which is responsible through the Secretary of State for Social Services, for health in England and for social security throughout the UK; the Scottish Home and Health

Department (again with more than one function), which reports through the Scottish Office to the Secretary of State for Scotland; the Welsh Office (with several functions) reporting to the Secretary of State for Wales; and the Department of Health and Social Services in Northern Ireland, which reports through the Northern Ireland Office to the Secretary of State for Northern Ireland (since the Northern Ireland Parliament ceased to exist).

Allocating money for the Health and Personal Social Services Programme is therefore more complicated than fixing the total expenditure of a single department. It is also worth noting that four Cabinet Ministers are involved in health policy, though three of them, as territorial ministers, are also responsible for services competing with health when resources are shared out. The Secretary of State for Social Services and the DHSS, however, take the lead in developing policy on health matters, and in the central discussions on allocation of funds. The allocations to the different countries of the UK are decided through the Public Expenditure Survey. We have mentioned the concern of the Health Departments that resources *within* each country should be allocated equitably, and we describe the approaches taken below. There has, however, been no attempt to provide an equitable basis for the allocation of resources as *between* the different countries. We take up this point in Chapter 8.

Resource Allocation by the Health Departments

Following reorganisation, the Health Departments asked working parties to produce methods to guide allocations towards an equitable and efficient response to relative needs. In England the DHSS asked the Resource Allocation Working Party (RAWP) to produce methods that could be used to guide the allocations of capital and revenue by the DHSS, regions and areas. In Scotland, Wales and Northern Ireland capital decisions are made by the Secretary of State in each country, and working parties in those countries considered the allocation of revenue only.

Resource Allocation in England

The RAWP was appointed in May 1975, produced an interim report in August 1975 and the final report in September 1976.[5] The Secretary of State announced that he would be broadly following the RAWP principles in allocating revenue budgets to Health Authorities in 1977—8. A year later, the method of the previous year was used to allocate *revenue* for 1978—9, and the Secretary of State announced that over the next few years a system of allocating *capital* would be introduced which would broadly follow the RAWP principles. The Secretary of State expected Health Authorities when allocating revenue to areas and districts to take account of the RAWP formula. The RAWP methods produce targets for revenue and capital against which current allocations can be compared. The general principle is that allocations ought to move towards these targets.

The revenue target of a Health Authority or District may have up to three components: two for service provision based on resident population and services provided for residents from other Authorities (or Districts); the third component is the Service Increment For Teaching (SIFT).

Figure 4.1 gives the build-up of the revenue target for service provision. (This is Figure II.4 of the RAWP Report with some minor amendments to bring it into line with current practice.) The overriding concept is an estimate of what resources would be allocated if the local resident population used resources at the same rate as the national average. For ambulance services and Family Practitioner Committee administration services the method simply multiplies the resident population by the national average expenditure per capita in England on those services. For services more directly concerned with health care this approach is too crude. The composition of the population crucially affects their relative needs for health care: for instance, elderly people and children have greater needs than adults between twenty and forty; and women and men also have different needs for care. Furthermore, the incidence of mental illness is higher among single than married people, and this factor is used to give a more sensitive estimate for mental care. The general approach for all day patients and out-patient services, mental illness in-patient services, mental handicap in-patient services, and for community services is to take national expenditure per capita in each relevant subgroup and multiply that by the number in the locality in that subgroup, and to sum these expenditures across the subgroups. For non-psychiatric in-patient services a more detailed approach is used. Here there is an attempt to identify the incidence of each condition according to the 17 chapter headings of the International Classification of Diseases (ICD). The surrogate measure used, is the Standardised Mortality Ratio (SMR), and for maternity care the Standardised Fertility Ratio (SFR). These ratios give for each age/sex and age group the actual rates as percentages of what they would be expected to be if the local occurrence were at the national average. The method first takes the number in each age/sex subgroup, and for each condition

Figure 4.1: The Build-up of the Revenue Target

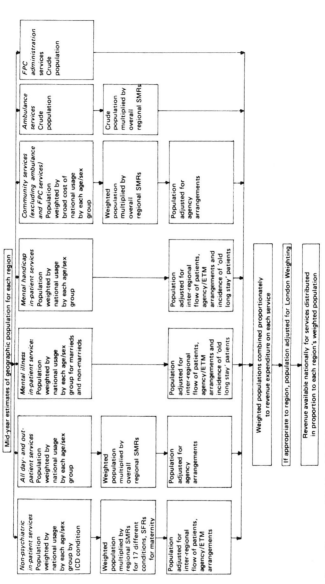

Mid-year estimates of geographic population for each region

Non-psychiatric in-patient services	All day- and out-patient services	Mental illness in-patient service:	Mental handicap in-patient services	Community services (excluding ambulance and FPC services)	Ambulance services	FPC administration services
Population weighted by national usage by each age/sex group by ICD condition	Population weighted by national usage by each age/sex group	Population weighted by national usage by each age/sex group for marrieds and non-marrieds	Population weighted by national usage by each age/sex group	Population weighted by broad cost of national usage by each age/sex group	Crude population	Crude population

| Weighted population multiplied by regional SMRs for 17 different conditions, SFRs for maternity | Weighted population multiplied by overall regional SMRs | | | Weighted population multiplied by overall regional SMRs | Crude population multiplied by overall regional SMRs | |

| Population adjusted for inter-regional flow of patients, agency/ETM arrangements | Population adjusted for agency arrangements | Population adjusted for inter-regional flow of patients, agency/ETM arrangements and incidence of 'old long stay' patients | Population adjusted for inter-regional flow of patients, agency/ETM arrangements and incidence of 'old long stay' patients | Population adjusted for agency arrangements | | |

Weighted populations combined proportionately to revenue expenditure on each service

If appropriate to region, population adjusted for London Weighting

Revenue available nationally for services distributed in proportion to each region's weighted population

Source: Department of Health and Social Security, *Sharing Resources for Health in England*, Report of the Resource Allocation Working Party (the RAWP Report) (HMSO, London, 1976), p. 26. Reproduced with the permission of the Controller of Her Majesty's Stationery Office.

multiplies this number by the relevant ratio (SMR or SFR), where appropriate, and by an estimate of the cost of treatment. These estimates of costs of treatment are then summed to give the local target component of non-psychiatric in-patient services.

The RAWP principle for capital allocation is to move towards equity of future *capital stock* in terms of relative need. The measurement of need for capital is directly analogous to that used in the revenue method. The resident population is again disaggregated into subgroups by age, sex, SMRs or SFRs and marital status as appropriate for the different services. The capital target is produced by taking the national capital stock per capita on each service within each population subgroup, multiplying this average by the local population of those subgroups, and summing across the subgroups and the different services. This method requires measures of capital stock, which is much more complicated than the analogous measure of revenue expenditure for the revenue target. There are two other differences from the revenue method. First, the population base is that predicted for five years ahead – the base for revenue calculations is most recent actual data. Second, the needs for capital for community care are treated differently from the revenue method, and weighted by GP consultation rates. FPC administration is omitted because it has minimal impact on capital requirements. The actual capital stock can then be compared with its target allocation.

In Chapter 8 we describe in more detail the approaches used in producing targets, particularly the use of SMRs as a proxy for morbidity, the difficulties of accounting for flow of patients across administrative boundaries, the problems of measuring capital stock, and the method used to value the SIFT.

Because the targets are only a rough guide the DHSS, in allocating revenue to regions, has to take into account important factors which are not easily quantified, as well as to judge the appropriate pace of movement towards equalisation. The DHSS advises regions and areas to make considered judgements about the pace of redistribution and to give greater weight to the unquantifiable factors because these become more important the smaller the size of the unit to which the allocation relates. For 1978–9 regions and areas were asked to notify the DHSS of the basis of their proposed allocations to areas and districts, and how these related to RAWP targets. Some regions have set up their own Resource Allocation Working Parties; and although the RAWP of the DHSS recommended that an area's allocation be built up from those of its constituent districts, a recent survey showed that this was exceptional in practice — it is common for districts' allocations to be made as subdivisions of area allocations.[6]

Part of the difficulty in making subregional allocations is in striking the balance between revenue and capital. Although the DHSS no longer grants money specifically for Revenue Consequences of Capital Schemes (RCCS), regions know that areas and districts need substantial extra revenue to fund capital developments when these are commissioned: new hospitals clearly create new demands on revenue, and even where the new hospital replaces an existing unit the newer services typically are significantly more expensive. Nine out of thirteen regions who replied to a recent questionnaire said that they had taken account of these revenue consequences in determining revenue targets for areas.[7]

Resource Allocation in Scotland

The Scottish equivalent of the RAWP — Scottish Health Authorities Revenue Equalisation (SHARE) — first met in March 1976 (after the submission of the RAWP's interim report) with the intention of making recommendations in time to guide resource allocation to Health Boards for 1977—8. The report comments that 'because of the complexity of the subject this time-scale proved to be unrealistic. . . an interim report was issued which made recommendations for minor adjustments to the present system of redistribution for 1977—78 only'.[8]

This interim report was submitted in September 1976 and all except two of its recommendations were accepted — those rejected related to limits on RCCS and on increases in allocations over the previous year. The final report was submitted in May 1977.

The Scottish working party considered the calculation of revenue targets only. These targets had the same components as in the RAWP approach although there are differences in the details of their calculation. The recommendations of the working party have been generally accepted by the Secretary of State for Scotland. They were used in the limited move made towards redistribution in 1978—9. Policy for the longer term was reviewed in 1978.

The working party recommended that the allocation of RCCS to Health Boards should be superseded, recognising that 'a modified form of financial assistance to take account of new developments will continue to be necessary'.[9] The assistance that has been introduced is that Health Boards will be able to 'bank' money with the SHHD in anticipation of heavy increases in future expenditure such as RCCS.

Resource Allocation in Wales

In Wales a working group on resource allocation was set up in 1974. This was superseded in 1976 by the Steering Committee on Resource Allocation.[10] This is a standing committee which makes recommendations to the Secretary of State for Wales on the allocation of capital (apart from major schemes) and revenue to areas. The committee uses a population-weighted formula which is refined each year. Because of the small populations and correspondingly small budgets of Welsh areas the extra revenue costs of new capital development cannot be accommodated without the assistance of RCCS by the Welsh Office. This practice is to be continued in Wales, and these grants use much of the increased growth money. Additional sums are also earmarked for funding in part the extra costs of new consultant appointments and improvements in services (in particular for the mentally ill and the mentally handicapped).

Resource Allocation in Northern Ireland

In Northern Ireland a working group on resource allocation first met in November 1977. Its terms of references were 'to recommend criteria for the allocation of revenue resources to Health and Social Service Boards in Northern Ireland, having regard to the recent reports on resource allocation in the National Health Service in Great Britain'. The report was published in November 1978, entitled *Proposals for the Allocation of Revenue Resources for Health and Personal Social Services* (the PARR Report).[12] It has been circulated for consultation and comment before the Secretary of State announces the basis on which future revenue will be related to the principles of the report. This working group had to deal with the smallest population of the countries of the UK (approximately 1.5 million). This is less than the smallest English region, and two of the four Boards are closer to the typical size of an English district as envisaged in the Grey Book (250,000) than to an area. Quantitative measures of need have to be used with considerable circumspection when allocation is on this reduced scale. Furthermore, Health Boards are also responsible for Personal Social Services, and so the working party had to go beyond the approaches used in the rest of the UK which consider health care only.

During the fieldwork for the Royal Commission the working party was just beginning. The Department of Health and Social Services – DHSS (NI) – allocated revenue on the basis of existing services, earmarked special expenditure on individual schemes, RCCS, and the remainder in blocks with broad directions on how this should be spent. Major capital decisions were taken by the department.

The remaining capital was allocated first to equipment and finally to minor schemes and associated equipment. The last of these was allocated to Boards in blocks on the basis of crude population.

Resource Allocation by English Health Authorities

The bulk of capital expenditure is decided at RHA level, after due process of consultation with AHAs and with the advisory committee structure and the DHSS. However, while capital spending in real terms has declined, revenue spending has increased moderately in real terms, and greatly in money terms (see Chapter 7), so that revenue spending currently represents some 90 per cent of total NHS expenditure.

Thus revenue spending dominates the NHS finances, and the bulk of revenue spending occurs at the level of areas and, especially, Health Districts. Successive reallocations of revenue funds must therefore be made; from RHA to AHA, AHA to district, and from district to the managers of its separate functional services.

Linking Budgeting to Resource Allocation

Historically, it appears that the NHS revenue-funds allocation process has been both incremental and iterative. It has been incremental in the sense that until recently there has been little budgetary challenge to the continued funding of the existing scale of established activities, and the allocation debate has been over the relative merits of alternative (incremental) uses of funds for new developments or the expansion of existing services – and over the related merits and urgency of competing claims from among the AHAs of a region, and the districts of an AHA. It has been iterative in the sense that even during the most generously-financed years of NHS expansion, the supply of finance has never met all demands, so that a process of consultation, referral and bargaining has been needed to scale down and match revenue demands to available funds. In good financial practice, budgets are viewed as much as a planning tool as a control tool. That is, budgets are not finalised until budget holders have reviewed their needs and put forward their requests for resources. Similarly, finance and or planning staff challenge the continued need for existing expenditure levels, and should assess the merit and economy of new budget requests from budget holders. Following reorganisation, a budgetary control system was introduced at each tier, so as to match expenditure accountability with the new functional management structure adopted in line with the the the Grey Book. The new budgetary system was called 'functional budgeting'.

Given that functional budgeting is still a new experience in the NHS (in some localities it has been in use for only two or three years) it is not surprising that often the budgets appear still to be operated more as a process of reallocation of funds, than as the positive budgetary management described above. This positive and interactive approach to budgeting seems likely to develop more strongly within the NHS in the years ahead, once greater experience of managing by budget is obtained, so long as undersized financial and planning teams are strengthened, and if greater realisation spreads that with a reduced rate of real growth in funds, an important portion of the funds for new developments must be found by challenging current expenditure and seeking savings therefrom.

The effective use of budgets in management requires that the senior holders of budgets (for particular services) should delegate management and accountability for relevant portions of their own budgets to their subordinates down the line of command. Budgetary delegation should match the degree of delegation of line authority over real resources – and the use of budgetary delegation and control should permit and encourage greater line-authority delegation. While staff have been adjusting to a new system there seems to have been some failure within many parts of the NHS to carry out both forms of delegation to a desirable degree. This may help to explain some of the delays and complexities of decision-making at the operational levels of the NHS, about which there has been so much complaint.

Budgetary Control and Clinical Autonomy

Budgetary control in the NHS has an important feature distinctively different from the typical practice in other public and private sector organisations. This is that the key front-line 'managers' in charge of hospital patient care do not themselves hold budgets or accept budgetary accountability. These 'managers' are the clinicians who have tended so far to feel that accepting responsibility for expenditure would conflict with their 'clinical autonomy'. It has been argued that this would involve a conflict of responsibilities between limiting total expenditure on resources for all their patients, and feeling duty bound to demand the use of all resources deemed needful for the care of individual patients. There is also a feeling that time spent on resource management and accounts is a waste of consultants' valuable training and skills.

It may be that a growing minority of clinicians are prepared to rethink their voluntary abstention from resource management and budgets. Certainly there are several experiments in progress around

Britain, where groups of clinicians are participating with finance officers and administrators in trials of specialty budgeting and specialty costing – two techniques that we discuss further in Chapter 11. Pending any future developments, however, one must be clear that budgetary management and accountability do not involve at present the clinicians who cause resources to be *consumed.* Instead, it is the managers of the various service functions – the *providers* of resources – who hold the budgets: this includes paramedical services, nursing, ambulance, catering, building and engineering, and general administration.

Notes

1. *National Loans Act 1968,* Ch. 13, section 12.

2. See *The Government's Expenditure Plans, 1979–80 to 1982–83,* Cmnd 7439 (HMSO, London, 1979), Tables 2.11, 4.5.1, 4.5.2 and 2.15.

3. The most recent is *The Government's Expenditure Plans, 1979–80 to 1982–83.*

4. See, for example, *Ninth Report from the Expenditure Committee, Session 1976–77,* Selected Public Expenditure Programmes, Ch. V: 'Spending on the Health and Personal Social Services' (HMSO, London, 1977).

5. Department of Health and Social Security (DHSS), *Sharing Resources for Health in England,* Report of the Resource Allocation Working Party (the RAWP Report) (HMSO, London, 1976).

6. National Association of Health Authorities, *Questionnaire on Resource Allocation* (June 1978).

7. Ibid.

8. Scottish Home and Health Department, *Scottish Health Authorities Revenue Equalisation (SHARE)* (HMSO, Edinburgh, 1977).

9. Ibid.

10. Welsh Office, *Report of the Steering Committee on Resource Allocation in Wales* (HMSO, Cardiff, 1976).

11. DHSS (Northern Ireland), *Proposals for the Allocation of Revenue Resources for Health and Personal Social Services,* Report of the Working Group on Revenue Resource Allocations to Health and Personal Social Services Boards in Northern Ireland, 1978 (the PARR Report).

12. Ibid.

5 PLANNING SYSTEMS

Following the 1974 reorganisation each Health Department intended to develop a framework for planning the development of health services based explicitly on the needs of patients. Formerly, planning had been primarily (though not exclusively) associated with the capital building programme. The general approach adopted in the UK, though with variations in Scotland, is to plan service development by care group. This approach, which classifies the need for services for different types of patients, has been designed so that planners can use the data produced by existing NHS information systems. The development of planning in each country of the UK has been different, both in the nature of the system adopted and the pace with which that system has been introduced.

The English system is the most ambitious attempt to introduce modern planning into the NHS. It consists of rolling three-year *operational* plans updated annually, and ten-year *strategic* plans updated every fourth year. English authorities are now producing the second cycle of strategic plans. Because this system is the most developed we concentrate on it, and use it as the basis for the review of planning problems in Chapter 9. Planning in England is of special interest because it is intended to mould policy on the bulk of NHS expenditure. Because of this ambitious aim, the English planning system is necessarily more complex than that introduced by other countries.

Planning in England
The Importance of Planning in the Making of Policy on Resources

In Chapter 3 we described the principles of the reorganised NHS in England. *Management Arrangements for the Reorganised National Health Service* (the Grey Book) set out six key features of the new arrangements which related directly to those principles. One of these features was 'Decentralisation of decision making, implicit in the patient-centred approach, can be balanced with the need for national and regional strategic direction by means of a planning system.'[1] The planning system which was introduced to provide this balance is described in *The NHS Planning System*. This emphasises the importance of planning: 'Members of Authorities as well as officials need personally to support and take part in planning because it is the single most important influence for better resource allocation.'[2]

Decisions on resource use in the reorganised NHS are to be informed by targets for allocations calculated by the RAWP principles and by policy on deployment formulated by the planning system. The targets for *allocation* provide the dynamic in moving the direction of capital and revenue towards need for care rather than in terms of past allocations. But how these financial resources are translated into service development to meet these changing needs is to be worked out by *planning*. And the planning system provides a means for monitoring the effects of redistribution of financial resources in terms of a more equitable access to services. It is worth clarifying how the methods of resource allocation, based on the principles of the RAWP (described in Chapters 4 and 8), and resource deployment, based on the planning system, are intended to work in harness. There is a vital difference between planning and resource allocation at the regional/DHSS interface and the use of the different systems subregionally.

In terms of the national policy on resources the DHSS uses the RAWP targets and makes judgements on the pace of movement towards equity between regions whose competing needs are not intended to be resolved through the planning system. The primary purpose of planning is to provide the system through which policy can be agreed between regions and the DHSS on how financial resources, once allocated, ought to be used.

Two points follow directly from this separation of planning from resource allocation at the DHSS/regional interface. First, the DHSS does not base its allocations on regional plans, and it is futile for regions to use this process to bid for resources beyond their likely allocations. Regions may believe that they need more money, but their need is a relative claim on limited resources. The DHSS makes these essentially national judgements relying on RAWP targets rather than plans. Second, regions can formulate policies which differ from those promulgated by the DHSS without putting their funding at risk. They are not completely free: the DHSS has controls over major capital expenditure and new consultant appointments, on which new developments often depend. As a way of influencing and monitoring regional policies on use of resources, however, these controls are less promising than using the planning system.

Subregionally, the systems of planning and resource allocation cannot sensibly be separated by regions and areas. The money to be allocated by regions to areas, for example, will depend on the plans approved for service development, which in turn must depend on regional policy decisions on relative needs, self-sufficiency and cross-boundary flows. There is need for continuing interplay between policies on resource allocation and on deployment — between dividing money geographically and deciding on the nature of service development — since the one depends on the other. A crucial element in the interplay is policy on the flow of patients across administrative boundaries. The RAWP methods do not of themselves provide a sound strategic basis for funding these flows. These strategic decisions can only be made through planning. We pursue this point in Chapter 8.

The Planning System — Guidelines and Plans

A brief authoritative outline of the NHS planning system is given in a note prepared by the DHSS for the Social Services and Employment Sub-Committee of the House of Commons Select Committee on Expenditure (the Expenditure Committee). This note explained that the system 'rests on the twin concepts of guidelines and plans'.[3] There are two kinds of guidelines and two levels of planning. The DHSS describes these, and how the guidelines and the different levels of planning relate to each other, as follows:

Two kinds of guidelines as issued by the Department to Regions and passed in turn to Areas and Districts:
(i) strategic guidelines concerned with general procedures and policies. The Consultative Documents on Priorities for Health and Personal Social Services in England (published in 1976) is an example.
(ii) operational guidelines drawn up specifically each year for the NHS operational planning process, indicating resource availability and priorities within that resource context.

Planning operates simultaneously on two levels as follows:
(i) strategic level — this is to devise broad strategies, priorities and resources for the period up to 10—15 years ahead; strategic plans are to be produced by Area Health Authorities (with the help of Districts) and by Regional Health Authorities every fourth year and reviewed annually. DHSS strategic planning provides an overall national framework.
(ii) operational level — here a sharper focus is taken by examining in detail action proposed for each of the next 3 years ahead — firm for year 1, provisional for year 2, and in outline for year 3. Three-year plans will be produced annually at District and Area

levels, with a Regional progress report, against the background of the strategic plans.

Plans will be reviewed by the next higher authority, and Regions will submit an annual report to the Department, thus completing the guidelines/planning cycle. Approval will not require or imply a positive endorsement of every proposal, or agreement with every judgement made by the planners. In principle, review is intended only to ensure that the plan generally accords with the guidelines and contains no feature to which the reviewing authority takes strong exception, or which is fundamentally inconsistent with other approved plans or is inadequate in any way. Any reservations by the reviewing authority will be taken into account in the next period.

In the light of its analysis of the Regional Strategic Plans, the Department will review the national strategies and priorities, and revise the guidelines for the subsequent year. There will be an analysis of expenditure by programme and sector (as in Annex 2 of the Consultative Document on Priorities) to provide a national picture of progress.[4]

Figure 5.1 gives a diagrammatic illustration of the relationships between guidelines and plans.

Strategic Planning

Further guidance on strategic planning was issued by the DHSS in a draft form in 1978 to help authorities to prepare the second round of strategic plans. This gives additional clarification of the purposes of strategic planning and of the different roles of regions and areas:

The function of *strategic planning* is:
(a) to identify a pattern of service provision, covering all aspects of the health authority's responsibilities, which on specified and realistic financial and manpower resource assumptions could be achieved within a period of ten years or thereabouts and which in the authority's view would best match the foreseen needs of the population served at that time: and
(b) to devise a strategy by which within the planning period the existing pattern of services could be transformed into that so identified.[5]

Regional Authorities have a major role to play in strategic planning. They have responsibility for financial allocations, major capital

Figure 5.1: The Flow of Guidelines and Plans in the NHS

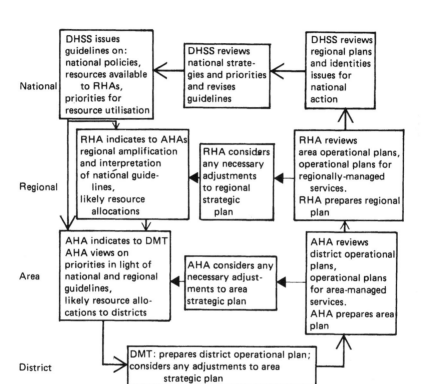

Source: Department of Health and Social Security, *The NHS Planning System* (HMSO, London, 1976), p. 10. Reproduced with the permission of the Controller of Her Majesty's Stationery Office.

projects and (except in teaching areas) consultant appointments. These key decisions will to a considerable extent determine the general directions of service development and deployment in the Region as a whole. The Regional Authority must therefore provide a strategic framework within which Areas can develop their own strategic plans. The Regional strategic framework should however itself be the subject of discussion with Area authorities. Discussion of the broad outline should precede the issue of Regional guidelines; when Areas have submitted plans within these guidelines, the Region can then firm up its own strategic plan, taking account of the problems and opportunities revealed by planned work at Area level.[6]

Operational Planning

Guidance on operational planning was given in *The NHS Planning System* and has not been added to. The publication described operational planning as:

the process by which decisions are reached on actual changes in service provision. . . In the main, it will be centred on the District. . . The operational plans of Districts generally will be based on proposals from planning teams which may be concerned with particular services or groups of services or other priorities determined locally, and from service managers. The particular point of the operational planning arrangements is that they must enable all proposals for change in the next three years, from whatever source, to be brought together and considered within a single structure, in order that the DMT may take a co-ordinated and comprehensive view of the whole District situation before deciding on particular proposals for change.[7]

Planning teams at district level were seen by the Grey Book as an important feature in the organisation of planning. The Grey Book named them Health Care Planning Teams (HCPTs) and suggested two types of team. One would be multidisciplinary and would bring together permanently those who work in hospitals (including consultants) and in the community (including social workers) to consider care groups which required this co-operation (e.g. the elderly, the mentally ill). The second type was temporary, and established to consider a particular problem. It was suggested that suitable projects would include studies within the acute care group (an example given was introduction of day surgery). These teams have been retitled District Planning Teams (DPTs).[8] A recent circular described the role of these teams as 'advisory and not executive'. Their functions are 'to develop, for the DMT, operational planning proposals within the general framework of AHA guidelines and to influence future strategies through commentary on these guidelines'.[9]

An Outline of Problems of Planning in England

Chapter 9 gives an extended review of planning in England. The purpose of this section is to give background information for that review by highlighting some of the problems.

Some Difficulties in Using the Care-group Approach

The eight care groups proposed by the DHSS are:

General and acute hospital services
Primary care services
Services mainly for the elderly and physically handicapped
Services for the mentally ill
Services for the mentally handicapped
Services mainly for children
Maternity services
Other

The classification of services by care group is given in *The NHS Planning System.*[10] There is, however, some scope for ambiguity in the assignment of services for the elderly. There has been a misconception that by making the development of these services a national priority the DHSS was advocating the development of long-stay care, whereas the Consultative Document pointed out that 'A modern geriatric service needs to provide for the direct admission of acutely medically ill elderly patients and in this aspect of its service does not differ from other acute specialties.'[11] The statistical distinction between acute/ elderly services depends on whether the care is administered under the supervision of a geriatrician (for example, in 1974, patients over 65 occupied 50 per cent of beds in general medicine and 39 per cent in general surgery[12]). Given the shortage of geriatricians, elderly people may receive the acute care that they need from general surgeons or general physicians, but this would not be classified as a service for the elderly.

A difficulty of using the care-group approach is that expenditure is not readily produced in the required form. The accounting and budgeting system disaggregates costs of hospitals by function (e.g. nursing, drugs, laundry), not by care group. It is nevertheless possible to derive approximate estimates of expenditure by care group.

Perhaps the most important weakness of the current definition of care group is the lumping together of all acute care within one block (which includes, *inter alia,* general medicine, general surgery, orthopaedic surgery, cardiology). This group of services accounts for 60 per cent of Health Authorities' expenditure. The current planning system gives no framework for setting priorities within this group.

Information for Planning

The difficulty of getting costs by care group is just one aspect of a general weakness of NHS information systems. The Grey Book criticised existing information for sometimes being 'unreliable, of doubtful relevance and out of date' and mentioned gaps especially on the needs of the community and the effectiveness of services in meeting these needs.[13] The RAWP Report commented:

A mass of information is collected regularly about NHS activities and facilities. Much of this is difficult to use to the full for allocation purposes because of problems in linking statistics from different data sources. Furthermore, despite the scale of the operation, important gaps still exist. Out-patients represent almost as large a proportion of NHS expenditure as all psychiatric patients, yet virtually nothing is known about their characteristics and movements. Community care, including family practitioner services, is a significant and increasing element in NHS provision, yet the data collected on these services fall far short in comprehensiveness and reliability of those on hospital in-patients.[14]

In February 1979 the DHSS issued a consultative document[15] on information requirements of the health service, following a preliminary study in 1978. The views of the NHS were characterised by 'widespread agreement that there should be changes in the substance of the data collected, the organisation of data collection and processing arrangements, and the attitude to be adopted on information matters generally'. Unfortunately, 'There was less agreement about how the process of change should be conducted and the pace at which it should take place.' The NHS was dissatisfied with the data now being collected because it was believed that they primarily served the interests of the department. This, it was suggested, had 'led to the work of collection being accorded a low priority and allocated to junior staff, sometimes without adequate supervision'. This problem was further exacerbated because the department's purposes for collecting data were not always clear to NHS staff. Not surprisingly the resulting malaise meant that even if the data were well designed for departmental purposes, 'much of the information provided was seen (by the Department) as being to some degree unreliable, inaccurate or incomplete', and 'Up-to-date information was often not available in time to help make important decisions.'

A NHS/DHSS steering group has been established to review proposals for change. Apart from basic virtues (such as timeliness, reasonable accuracy and avoiding duplication) the guiding principles are based on local needs, compatibility and relating data to identifiable purposes. Whilst the planning system and the RAWP methods both highlight weaknesses in current data and point the way to kinds of data which are relevant to informed decision-making, there is an organisational weakness which may well hinder this necessary development.

The two key roles in planning are those of the administrator and the community physician. (By community physician we mean the specialist who is a member of management teams or teams of officers: i.e. the District Community Physician (DCP), the Area Medical Officer (AMO) and the Regional Medical Officer (RMO).) The community physician is expected to take the lead in the formulation of plans of services directly concerned with health care. The administrator is expected to co-ordinate and implement these plans and discharge each of these tasks for supporting services. In terms of information, the community physician is responsible for improving data on health care: but staff shortages make this difficult (see below), and the staff who collect the data report up the administrative line. The whole management team was given general responsibility for data (by the Grey Book), but the failure to vest responsibility clearly with one role (together with the necessary staff) was identified in our report[16] as a major impediment to improvement. This point is not however made by the DHSS in the most recent circular.

The Difficulties of the Community Physician

The Grey Book proposed a management structure which depended to a considerable extent on well-qualified staff in community medicine. At area and regional levels, posts were created for Specialists in Community Medicine (SCMs). These staff were intended to provide support not only for AMOs and RMOs but also for the DCPs. One of the key responsibilities assigned to the community physician was the formulation of plans for services directly concerned with the provision of health care. This was only one of a formidable list of tasks assigned to community physicians.

The burden of work assigned to staff in community medicine was described by the Kogan Report:

The roles of area/regional medical officer and district community physician were thought by their role holders to contain what could easily be two full time posts: medical administration and specialists in community medicine. Besides administration, the planning function of community medicine implied an increased level of research and data refinement which would lead to evaluation of services and modification of priorities among services. This aspect of community medicine was largely overlooked because few community physicians were able to avoid the demands of medical administration, including a great deal of work with hospitals, which took up the community physician's allocation of time.[17]

The problem of discharging these important planning tasks will become more severe. This is because many staff in post will be retiring over the next few years. There are already serious shortages of suitably qualified staff — many posts in community medicine have remained vacant.

Recruits to community medicine are not sufficiently numerous to make good the prospective losses from retirement. This problem is so severe that it is seen as requiring central direction. A DHSS circular, *Review of Management Costs,* commented on community medicine posts in these terms:

> It has . . . become clear that the losses which can be expected from retirement and other causes among existing filled posts up to 1980 exceed even an optimistic projection of the number of suitably qualified doctors who can be recruited in the same period . . . the numbers of posts filled nationally can be expected to fall appreciably below present levels. The incidence of losses is bound to occur in an irregular pattern geographically and there are risks that some Regions or Areas might find themselves unable to fill essential functions in the community medicine field. For these reasons the Secretary of State has decided that control of community medicine establishments and vacancies for each Region must be exercised centrally by the Department with the advice of the Manpower Advisory Committee (Community Medicine).[18]

The community physician has been given a difficult role in planning services directly concerned with health care. To be successful he must gain the respect of clinicians. This is of itself difficult to achieve because clinicians tend to be grudging in respecting doctors who are administrators and who no longer treat patients. If the efficient planning of health services means anything to clinicians — and we cannot believe the contrary — it must be that respect can still be won by demonstration of the ability to present a clearly argued case based on both medical understanding and on a wide grasp of conditions outside the hospital, and of national and local policies.

Staff shortages are likely to mean that community physicians will not have the necessary support or time to discharge properly all their duties and to win the respect of clinicians by demonstration of expertise in planning for the community. An issue of particular importance is the development of acute care (which accounts for 60 per cent of Health Authorities' expenditure). Hospital doctors are a powerful and influential group in decisions on acute care. National guidance on the balance across care groups gives little direction within acute care, and the available data are also inadequate for informed debate. We pursue this issue in Chapter 9. The relevant background described here is how clinicians are involved in planning.

Clinicians and Planning

The Grey Book laid great emphasis on clinical involvement. One of the aims of reorganisation was to promote 'Means whereby doctors and dentists can contribute more effectively to NHS decision making.'[19] One of the five principles was that 'health-care professions should be integrally involved in planning and management at all levels'.[20] Despite this last principle, the Grey Book focused clinical involvement at district level because 'The District is the largest-sized unit within which consultants, general practitioners and others can participate actively in the management process through effective representative systems.'[21] And it is worth noting that, although clinical involvement in multi-district areas and regions through Area/Regional Medical Advisory Committees was seen by the Grey Book as 'an important means by which local clinicians can be consulted by the Area and Regional Authorities and their officers on crucial planning issues', the Grey Book states that 'the structure and functions of medical advisory committees do not directly concern the management study'.[22]

In the Grey Book, districts were responsible for operational and strategic planning. When the planning system was introduced, areas and regions were made responsible for strategic planning, and operational planning was made primarily a district responsibility. Thus in multi-district areas the formulation of strategy takes place at a level previously thought to be inappropriate for the adequate involvement of clinicians. And the Grey Book, of course, did not consider how clinical involvement should take place within the current planning system. We review in this section the proposals made by the Grey Book for clinical involvement, and discuss in Chapter 9 the difficulties of securing this involvement in strategic planning.

The District Management Team includes three doctors: the District Community Physician, a consultant and a general practitioner. These last two are representatives of clinicians, being elected by the District Medical Committee (DMC). The Grey Book says that this committee, which 'should represent all general practitioners and hospital doctors and co-ordinate the medical aspects of health care throughout the District, should be fairly small, usually about a dozen'.[23] The Grey Book stresses that the DCP is not expected 'to give clinical advice and is not empowered to speak for clinicians'.[24] The consultant and general practitioner are expected to do this but the Grey Book draws attention to two limitations of their roles in management. First, they 'are active clinicians and their continuing credibility as representatives rests on this fact. They will therefore be able to spare only part of their time for the business of the DMC and the DMT'.[25] Second, 'they take their places not as heads of hierarchically-organised professions but as elected representatives of equals'.[26] Despite these limitations, the Grey Book expected them to 'enjoy the confidence of their colleagues, so that they can speak for clinicians not as mere delegates, unable to commit their peers without reference back, but as representatives using the discretion vested in them as a basis for action'.[27]

The Kogan Report considered the role of clinicians in management, and commented: 'The somewhat bland assertions of the reorganisation documents that clinicians will take part in team discussions and be full partners in consensus management understate the considerable novelty and difficulties of this role.'[28] The *Report of the Committee of Inquiry into Normansfield Hospital* was concerned about the difficulty and ambiguity of the role of the consultant member of the management team, and pointed to the importance of clarifying his responsibilities and those of the community physician.[29] Of particular concern, given the general theme of this book, is the lacuna identified by the Kogan Report:

> At a time of limited funds, the tension between professional ideals and accountable management becomes sharper because it is less easy to meet individual demands, but the relationship of doctors to management structure, in their individual roles as practitioners, as representatives of other doctors and as members of management teams, is still far too unclear.[30]

The Kogan Report did note a variety of models of clinician involvement ranging from roles of representative to delegate. Trouble had occurred in one team because the consultant member had agreed to a team decision with which the area's consultants strongly disagreed. The Area Medical Advisory Committee passed a vote of no confidence in its representative, who was replaced. His successor 'was very conscious of the limitations of acceptability which the medical staff might place on management team decisions'.[31] The general concern about the medical advisory structure is that by focusing on overcoming the weaknesses of the tripartite structure of 1948, it does not seem to be equipped for resolving the difficult issues of rationing hospital services we now face.

Organisational Structure and Planning

Single-district areas do conform to the Grey Book's concept of planning. Unfortunately this does not mean that they are better equipped to discharge their planning responsibilities. These authorities have three demanding jobs to do. First, they have to run the health services of a district for a population of approximately 200,000 (and in some cases 500,000). Second, each year they have to roll forward an operational plan. Third, every fourth year they have to produce a strategic plan. However, strategic planning is intended to be a process and should be a continuous activity.

The two single-district areas we visited found it difficult to do all these tasks properly: they did not seem to be adequately staffed. The Grey Book's proposal that to have all three tiers of the NHS prepare operational and strategic plans does not seem sensible. The current structure, which has vested responsibility for strategic planning at only two levels (areas and regions), has still encountered problems. Regions have to take a strategic view on capital development before they can give resource guidelines to areas. This view is best informed by areas' strategic plans. These plans cannot be produced without guidelines from the region on future resources.

Planning in Wales

The planning system introduced by the Welsh Office at the same time as the DHSS in England has some similarities with the English system. There are, however, important differences in that formal responsibility for the production of plans is vested with areas only, and the system is still evolving in terms of the production of operational and strategic plans. We begin by describing the organisation of planning, and conclude this section with a description of how the system has been developing.

Organisation for Planning

Although the Welsh Office, in planning for Wales, faces responsibilities similar to those of an RHA in addition to those of a government department, current policy is to limit the Welsh Office's formal contribution to planning, to guidance to areas on policies and resources: there is no intention to draw together plans produced by areas into an all-Wales plan. Districts in Wales have no formal responsibility for producing plans. They can contribute to planning by the work of District Planning Teams. Areas are responsible for the production of both operational and strategic plans. But, as we explain below, there is no similar cycle for the production of these plans in Wales as in England.

The Developing Welsh Planning System

Capital development is a major component of strategic planning. The Secretary of State is responsible for deciding the programme of major capital work, and has made a number of decisions which will be executed over the next ten years. Decisions have still to be taken during this period on other major developments. Some of the decisions on capital have been taken outside the planning system, but it is intended that future capital proposals should emerge from that system. It is hoped to announce a programme of intermediate capital development. These decisions, together with guidance on priorities, should provide the necessary strategic framework for planning by areas.

The Welsh Office have promulgated priorities[32] and published a Service Planning Series of papers to guide area planning. In the first round (1976–7) areas were asked to produce plans for the short term 'against the context of a brief outline of the objectives and priorities of each client or service group in medium (3–10 years) and long term (10–15 years)'.[33] Not all areas had completed these plans before the second cycle was launched. Because of this unequal response and because of the mixed quality of those plans received (which tended to be weak on policy for the short term), the Welsh Office asked for different plans in the second cycle according to the stage of planning achieved by areas. For 1977–8 those areas with a satisfactory planning framework were asked to produce a shorter operational planning statement in 1977. Areas that had yet to produce a full strategic plan were asked to prepare one for 1977–8 along the lines proposed for 1976–7. Areas were asked to relate their 1978 operational plans to strategic objectives where these had already been identified, or to indicate specifically the strategic context in which it was placed (where these objectives had not been identified or had changed). The Welsh Office further expressed an intention to review the planning process in order to secure improvements in the quality and utility of plans. This process is continuing.

Planning in Scotland

In the early years following reorganisation the effort was directed towards first, the development of the strategic planning system, particularly the departmental phase of the strategic planning cycle, and second, the establishment of an advisory structure to assist policy-making at the centre. We begin by describing the advisory system.

Organisation for Central Policy-Making in Scotland

The Scottish Health Service Planning Council (SHSPC). The SHSPC consists mainly of one member of each of the Health Boards and medical schools, together with officers of the Scottish Home and Health Department (SHHD). It works through advisory groups of two kinds. First, there are *ad hoc* groups, mostly programme planning groups which prepare reports on particular subjects. Second, there are more permanent advisory groups which give technical advice as required on, for instance, information and computer services, and blood transfusion. These groups advise the Planning Council, which in turn gives advice to the Secretary of State. The permanent advisory groups, like the National Consultative Committees discussed in the next paragraph, may also in some instances advise the Secretary of State directly.

National Consultative Committees (NCCs). Seven NCCs have been formed and are now the principal source of advice from professions who provide health care. They naturally give advice on matters referred directly to them. They are also involved in planning: they give professional and technical advice to programme planning groups of the SHSPC; draft reports from these groups go to the relevant NCCs for comment; and the chairmen of the NCCs are invited to attend SHSPC meetings.

The Organisation of Planning in the Scottish Health Boards

As in Wales (but not as in England), districts have not been given planning responsibilities. Health Boards have established interdisciplinary groups for planning by care group known as Programme Planning

Groups (PPGs). These are similar to the English and Welsh District Planning Teams in membership but they are organised at Board (not district) level. PPGs are intended to carry out detailed investigations of a few fields which appear important enough to justify the staff input. They will be wound up on completion of the work.

One of the problems facing these PPGs is that they are not backed by a formal planning process, so that they cannot look towards a clear statement of Board policies. The Board we visited had attempted to overcome this omission. A statement of national priorities was issued by the Secretary of State in April 1976 in order to give Health Boards guidance as to how the expenditure restrictions announced at the time were to be implemented. Because of the urgency only limited consultation with the SHSPC was possible. This was published as *The Health Service in Scotland − The Way Ahead.*[34] The Board had attempted to follow these priorities by an analysis of ·expenditure by care group, but since there was no mechanism for regular review it was difficult to know whether progress was being made. The Board had also published in draft both short and long-term plans for consultation. Despite these attempts to formulate a longer-term direction, the Board's main emphasis was on the details of operational management.

The Planning Unit of SHHD has developed proposals for a strategic planning system which have been accepted by SHSPC. The proposed system is intended to be both simple and flexible, to unify planning at area and central levels, and to encourage decentralised decision-making. The planning cycle, which may take five years to complete, would begin with the department undertaking a thorough review of its own work, and preparing national guidelines. These would indicate the priority to be given to each programme, and the financial resources likely to be available. They would then be used by Health Boards to perform a similar review of their own activities and to produce an area planning statement setting priorities and objectives for their own areas. The 15 area planning statements would be combined into a composite planning statement setting priorities and objectives for consideration by the Planning Council and the SHHD, and for use in the next departmental review. Wide-ranging consultations would take place at national level on the proposed national guidelines, and at Board level on draft area planning statements.

Planning in Northern Ireland

As we have mentioned in Chapter 3, the reorganised NHS in Northern Ireland (introduced on 1 October 1973) included personal social services as a responsibility of the newly constituted Health Boards. One of the underlying concepts of management of the Health and Personal Social Services were 'programmes of care' defined in terms of resources directed towards a care group. The DHSS (NI) issued general policies to Health Boards in January 1974. This guidance included tables similar to those of the DHSS on guidelines of provision by care group, in terms of staffing and beds in relation to the appropriate population. (A point of interest is that these guidelines do disaggregate the acute care group by specialty. The total for the group is 3.5 beds/thousand population whereas the English guideline is 3 beds/thousand appropriate population.)

In 1975, after consultation with the Health and Social Services Council and the Boards, the DHSS (NI) published its strategy for service development.[35] The priorities of this strategy are similar to those of the other countries in the UK (e.g. emphases on community care, the elderly, the mentally ill, the mentally handicapped). These priorities include development of teaching and research, and improvements in information systems. The strategy was to be implemented by planning by the DHSS (NI) and the Boards on the basis of programmes of care. The published strategy outlined a seven-stage planning process, and explained that it would be further elaborated in detailed guidance and a series of papers on the development of programmes of care.

At the time of our research in late 1977/early 1978 the DHSS (NI) had still not issued the papers promised in 1975. But planning was still being attempted and one Board had submitted a plan to the department. As part of our study the Northern Ireland research team interviewed staff and members in one of the Boards, which had not yet produced an area plan. Two points emerged which are of general significance, given the differences between Northern Ireland and England. First (and perhaps most obviously, given the lack of guidance on planning issued by the department since the publication of its strategy), there was considerable confusion about the planning system within the Board. More than half of those interviewed either denied or were unaware of the existence of an annual planning cycle. Second, the Programme Planning Teams exclude clinicians. This omission was seen as one of the reasons why none of the four teams established had been able to produce a programme of care. The Board attempted to produce a plan without these programmes, and instead had to rely on departmental guidelines, needs identified by pressure on services, and professional judgements.

In May 1978 a seminar was held to promote a new planning system.

It had become clear that the seven-stage process outlined in 1975 was not working and that the only effective planning taking place was in capital development. Following that meeting a discussion paper was circulated which suggested that the Scottish approach was probably most appropriate for Northern Ireland. It was hoped to launch a re-vamped planning system in 1979.

Notes

1. Department of Health and Social Security (DHSS), *Management Arrangements for the Reorganised National Health Service* (the Grey Book) (HMSO, London, 1972), p. 11.

2. DHSS. *The NHS Planning System* (HMSO, London, 1976), p. 5.

3. *Ninth Report from the Expenditure Committee.* Session 1976–7, Selected Public Expenditure Programmes, Ch. V: 'Spending on the Health and Personal Social Services' (HMSO, London), p. 2.

4. Ibid., pp. 2–3.

5. DHSS, *Draft Addendum to The NHS Planning System. Future Form and Content of Strategic Plans,* issued with a covering letter from Mr R. S. King to Regional Administrators, 11 January 1978, p. 1.

6. (Ibid.) p. 4.

7. DHSS, *NHS Planning System*, p. 15.

8. DHSS, *Joint Care Planning: Health and Local Authorities,* Health Circular HC (77) 17/Local Authority Circular LAC (77) 10 (May 1977).

9. DHSS, *DHSS Planning Guidelines for 1978/79.* Health Circular HC (78) 12 (March 1978).

10. DHSS, *NHS Planning System*, p. 52.

11. DHSS, *Priorities for Health and Personal Social Services in England*, A Consultative Document (HMSO, London, 1976), p. 40.

12. DHSS, *The Way Forward* (HMSO, London, 1977), p. 19.

13. Grey Book, p. 55.

14. DHSS, *Sharing Resources for Health in England*, Report of the Resource Allocation Working Party (the RAWP Report) (HMSO, London, 1976), p. 82.

15. DHSS, *Management Services – Information Requirements of the Health Services,* HN (79) 21 (February 1979).

16. *Management of Financial Resources in the National Health Service,* Royal Commission on the National Health Service, Research Study No. 2 (HMSO, London, 1978), p. 60.

17. *The Working of the National Health Service* (the Kogan Report), Royal Commission on the National Health Service, Research Study No. 1 (HMSO, London, 1978), p. 43.

18. DHSS, *Health Services Management – Review of Management Costs,* HC (77) 10 (April 1977).

19. Grey Book, p. 10.

20. Ibid.

21. Ibid., p. 13.

22. Ibid., p. 70.

23. Ibid., p. 68.

24. Ibid., p. 70.

25. Ibid., p. 69.

26. Ibid.

27. Ibid.

28. Kogan Report, p. 70.

29. *Report of the Committee of Inquiry into Normansfield Hospital*, Cmnd 7357 (HMSO, London, 1978), p. 384.

30. Kogan Report, p. 71.

31. Ibid., p. 67.

32. Welsh Office, *Proposed All-Wales Policies and Priorities for the Planning and Provision of Health and Personal Social Services from 1976–77 to 1979–80* (HMSO, Cardiff, 1976).

33. Welsh Office, *Service Planning 6, Format of Area Plans 1976/77* (HMSO, Cardiff, 1976).

34. Scottish Home and Health Department, *The Health Service in Scotland – The Way Ahead* (HMSO, Edinburgh, 1976).

35. DHSS (Northern Ireland), *Strategy for the Development of Health and Personal Social Services in Northern Ireland, 1975.*

6 MONITORING AND CONTROL

Parliamentary Accountability

Parliament monitors the management of the NHS through two processes. The first is the traditional one whereby the minister (or, for the NHS, the Secretary of State) is accountable to Parliament. This accountability focuses on his ability to answer for apparent shortcomings through parliamentary questions. The second process is comparatively recent and is an extension of the Expenditure Committee's examination of the Government's expenditure plans: a subcommittee examines the DHSS on the programme for Health and Personal Social Services.

The nature of ministerial responsibility. is not straightforward: of course the minister does not know in advance that a junior clerk is going to make a damaging decision on somebody's pension, or muddle up an admission into hospital; and of course he does not authorise the clerk's decision in advance, not knowing the detail of the case. But this does not exonerate him from responsibility for what has happened; his job is to run his department in such a way that agreed policies get applied and so that his staff do *not* make damaging mistakes — at least, not in circumstances where the organisation or attitude of the department is at fault. And the minister's responsibility does not mean that the clerk is not also responsible to his superiors; and indeed all the intermediate managers below the Secretary of State (like those in any hierarchical organisation) are answerable to their superiors for what happens in their sphere of responsibility, whether or not they know about detailed decisions in advance.

This is a little different if the organisation is not entirely hierarchical — e.g. when it includes professionals acting as such, and when semi-autonomous tiers are interposed. The minister is still answerable for the way his powers have been used, and for the general level and quality of services which have been provided by doctors and health authorities. There is a difficult and delicate line to be drawn between the cases on which a minister will or will not be expected to answer. The reader may like to consider what answer the minister should give to the following questions:

a. 'Why did Doctor A give Mrs M treatment X instead of Y?'
b. 'Why did Doctor A admit Mrs M rather than Mrs N?'

   c. 'On what grounds are patients selected from the waiting list in
     area G for treatment X?'
   d. 'Is the minister satisfied with the long and increasing waiting list
     in area G for treatment X while there are spare beds in depart-
     ment Z in the same area?'

The minister will certainly answer a. to the effect that this is a matter
for the individual clinician. He may seek to do the same on b., but this
aspect is becoming more a matter of public policy, and if he declines
to give a substantive answer he can be asked c.: and an MP worth his
salt would not be content with an answer which laid entire responsibility on the clinician or on the managing authority. Similarly, a minister might be unwise to dodge question d., which is a matter of proper
public concern, although the minister may, of course, reply that he is
satisfied and explain why. This explanation may rest on his acceptance
of clinical judgement. If the NHS were an autonomous corporation like
the Post Office became in 1972, many more questions could properly
be declined on the grounds that this was the responsibility of the
Health Authority in question. This might be convenient for authorities,
but not so good for the public: apart from anything else, Health Departments would not be able to give directions on national policies or
priorities, nor to check how services were being administered.

    We elaborate this point not so much because of the obvious con-
flict between answerability for others and personal clinical or nursing
responsibility, but because there is a need for a wider understanding
of the manner in which ministers are in fact responsible for the way
their powers have been used (or not used), and for the services and the
results which have been provided (or have been deficient or perhaps
refused). This is particularly important when (as we emphasise elsewhere in this book) resources are likely to fall short of those which
are demanded for health care.

    In some circumstances there may be further responsibilities on
top of those we have enumerated − to the Courts, who may hold that
the terms of an Act of Parliament oblige the Secretary of State and his
officers to provide certain services: they may also, of course, occasion-
ally hold that he has taken action which was outside his powers.

    The mainstream responsibility, however, which permeates depart-
mental life at various levels, is financial responsibility. The minister
is responsible, in particular for the results of allocating and using
money in one way rather than another, and for doing so efficiently
or inefficiently, and therefore for ensuring that his subordinates with
delegated powers know enough of the results of central decisions on

policy, or on resource allocation, for their decisions to be taken in an informed and rational manner.

Monitoring through the Planning System

In the first report of the subcommittee of the Expenditure Committee into the Health and Personal Social Services Programme, a witness from the DHSS explained that the planning system is the means through which the DHSS can try to convey to the subcommittee 'the product of a year's work and the deployment of a year's money.'[1] The witness suggested that the opportunities for reporting personally in this way to Parliament were limited outside the new procedures of the Select Committee: the traditional means of questions and answers in the House and parliamentary debate, were less apt for examining the development of the NHS.

Annual Planning Reports

Regional Annual Planning Reports (APRs) provide the direct means by which the DHSS intends to link parliamentary accountability to Health Authorities' progress in implementing regional strategies agreed with the DHSS. The regional strategic plan, as approved by the DHSS, enables each RHA to agree strategies of its constituent AHAs which are consistent with departmental policies. Districts are the level at which operational planning begins: these plans are intended to set out three-year rolling programmes through which the area strategy is to be implemented. The APRs describe progress made in implementing the strategy.[2]

The quality of monitoring through the planning system depends crucially on the quality of the planning process. The first round of strategic plans (produced in 1976–7) were generally unsatisfactory, and tended to be particularly weak on costing and in considering uncertainty. The main purposes of planning ought to be agreeing priorities and developing a robust strategy of implementing those priorities. Plans formed in this way provide a sound basis for monitoring developments against what was planned. Plans which are weak in these respects may be difficult to relate to what happens: for example, one should be aware of deviations from the plan early enough to modify or abandon it, rather than attempt to force developments to take the planned direction. The second round of strategic plans are a significant improvement on the earlier attempts, and one consequence should be that monitoring will become more effective.

Relating Planning to Financial Controls

It is vital that monitoring through the planning system be developed because the primary controls inherited from before the planning system was introduced are of a limited kind. We discuss these below. They focus on expenditure against a budget, and on the propriety of that expenditure. The important issues of whether the agreed budgets are appropriate are not examined by these systems. Apart from the need to develop reporting of achievement — which APRs are intended to provide — there is the question of linking expenditure to plans. This is not straightforward because budgets are controlled by function, whereas plans are drawn up in terms of care groups. At this stage it is not clear how these two can best be linked.

One approach would be to develop the accounting system to report expenditure by care group. The expenditure could then be monitored during the year against the operational plan. Without this link there can be delays in examining the pattern of expenditure and relating this to the plan. Consider for example an operational plan for three financial years beginning in 1980—1. The actual expenditure by care group for that year will, given current systems, not be estimated until after the financial year 1981—2 has begun and the plans for the three-year period beginning with that year have been produced. Discrepancies between what was planned and what happened during 1980—1 could therefore only begin to be corrected in the plans for 1982—3, and whether this action had been successful would not be known until 1983—4.

The process of monitoring is inseparable from planning, and appropriate developments in financial reporting depend upon the nature of operational planning. If operational planning becomes a comprehensive review (and in Chapter 12 we suggest a development of this kind as one of a number of changes) then it may be sensible to develop the accounting system to provide comprehensive, up-to-date expenditure by care group. If, however, strategic planning provides the comprehensive overview and operational planning picks out a small set of targets then operational plans are best monitored in terms of achievement of those targets, rather than by a comprehensive accounting system.

Annual Accounting Reports

Health Districts and Authorities prepare annual accounts on an 'income and expenditure' basis of accounting, for review at the next tier, and transmission upwards to the DHSS.[3] Whilst these annual accounts report interesting and indeed useful information, and even though they are studied carefully at the DHSS, they have not been used to the full because they are out of date by the time they are available. Other sources of more up-to-date information have had to be developed. The DHSS (and Treasury) obtain the financial information they most need from monitoring the health authorities reports under FIS (HA) (Financial Information System, Health Authorities), and from the Treasury FIS, which works on records of cash payments by departments, including issues to Health Authorities. Moreover the annual accounts (like many other public-sector accounts) provide very little information concerning capital-asset values and the cost of capital resources consumed, or concerning the impact of inflation upon resource consumption in real terms.

Certain standard categories of cost information are also collected and reported to the DHSS by Health Authorities. Once again, we understand the value of this information is limited by the delay in its publication, and because inflation has overtaken the relevance of the information by the time it is made available for comparative study. In our discussions with NHS treasurers, many of them felt that the present form of cost classification does not provide them with useful information, and that scarce financial manpower is better employed in trying to make functional budgeting work, rather than in trying to expedite or interpret the presently available cost information. If specialty costing (see Chapter 11) can be made to work, then there may become available a form of cost information more valuable for planning than the present functional cost information, for both central planning at the DHSS, and operational planning and management at local level.

Control by Functional Budgets

Below the level of the individual Health Districts and Authorities, the detailed monitoring and control of revenue expenditure must be achieved through budget holders, supported by finance officers, maintaining up-to-date scrutiny of expenditure as compared to authorised budget.[4] This should involve prompt and error-free reporting of expenditure against budget for every budget-holding manager. Our own researches have shown that as recently as early 1978 budgetary performance reports were often supplied to budget holders undesirably late, and errors were too numerous. In addition, comprehensive budget reports should include existing financial commitments, not just actual expenditure, in order to provide a realistic picture of the funds remaining and available for spending within the budget limits. The typical NHS functional budget systems in current use do not include such commitment accounting.

The obvious reason for the technical shortcomings of current budgetary control procedures is the newness of the present systems. Important contributory factors must be the shortage (relative to the size of organisations involved) of experienced middle-grade and senior accounting and finance staff, and also the lack of facilities and sufficient trained staff for full computerisation of budget information. The control and cutback on management costs in the NHS, apparently to be reinforced by the new Government, makes it difficult to remedy staff shortages quickly; but there are hopeful indications that in future the DHSS will allow AHAs and Health Districts to acquire greater computer power under their own control, instead of having to rely mainly on often unsatisfactory relationships with RHA mainframe computer-service organisations. Computing needs good software as well as hardware, of course, and with DHSS support the West Midlands RHA has been developing and pilot-testing programmes known as the Standard Accounting System (SAS). The SAS reportedly shows promise, includes a commitment accounting facility, and should be capable of general adoption and of providing faster and more accurate budgetary control reports and summaries, including information on specialty costs and specialty budgets. More recently, a research programme (to report in autumn 1980 and autumn 1981) has been mounted by West Midlands RHA with DHSS support. It is to investigate the financial information required in support of health care planning, and by clinicians in the organisation and management of their units, and to design, develop and implement systems for its production.

In spite of the shortcomings in the present systems of reporting and monitoring expenditure by individual budget holders (which we discuss further in Chapter 11), it appears from our enquiries that most NHS budget holders have in fact managed to keep within their budgets, so that relatively few authorities have been embarrassed by net overspending. Of course, the fact that 75 per cent or more of many budget allocations consists of salaries and wages, whose rates (and numbers of staff allowed) for the year were known at the time of budget setting, does make budget compliance easier. Also, many budget holders operate their own informal systems of recording orders and commitments, and these informal systems have compensated for the reporting delays and other shortcomings of the formal budgetary control system.

In the infrequent cases where a budget holder wilfully and needlessly overspends his budget, the typical drill appears to be as follows. First, the Finance Officer supplies advice and pressure, and the budget holder's local line superior and the local administrator may also become involved. If all this fails to rectify budgetary performance, the matter may then be formally considered by the local management team or officer team, or even be referred to the Health Authority itself. We understand, however, that it is rare for this further stage of budgetary discipline to be needed, or used.

Internal and External Audit

Like other substantial organisations, the NHS is subject to both internal audit and external audit.[5] Each Health Authority has its own internal audit team; although, as we have elsewhere explained in greater detail, we think that insufficient resources and status have been conferred upon internal audit in the NHS, so that its performance as an aid to monitoring and control — especially on matters of efficiency and effectiveness as distinct from basic stewardship and probity audits — in many but not all authorities lags well behind the standards attained frequently in well-managed private concerns and other public authorities. Similarly, we have criticised the DHSS for, until recently, failing to give sufficient priority to high-grade recruitment and training for its own staff of auditors, who provide the external audit services to the NHS.[6] Additionally the NHS is subject to special audits by staff of the Comptroller and Auditor General. These latter audits are deemed to be highly competent, but they are linked to parliamentary interests in the use of funds, and it appears to us that they have limited impact on the operational-level management of the NHS.

Conclusion

This chapter has been brief. It has been brief because, whilst there exists in the NHS a fairly typical public-sector system of monitoring the amount and probity of expenditure, the arguably more important aspects of monitoring (and control) barely exist as yet. These aspects are concerned with measuring performance in resource-use efficiency and effectiveness. They depend upon comparing performance against plans: as NHS planning improves, better monitoring should (and can) be developed to make this comparison possible. We discuss further, in Chapter 11, some particular problems of NHS financial control, and developments that might improve monitoring and control.

Notes

1. *Ninth Report from the Expenditure Committee,* Session 1976–7, Selected Public Expenditure Programmes, Ch. V: 'Spending on the Health and Personal Social Services' (HMSO, London, 1977), Q. 265.

2. See *Management of Financial Resources in the National Health Service,* Royal Commission on the National Health Service, Research Paper, No. 2 (HMSO, London, 1978), pp. 74–6.

3. Ibid., pp. 130–2.

4. Ibid., pp. 102–6.

5. Ibid., pp. 158–65.

6. Ibid., p. 165.

7 THE COST OF SPENDING MORE

The Scale of Expenditure on Health Services

Public expenditure on health services (excluding personal social services) in 1979–80 is programmed at rather over £7,200m at the prices of autumn 1977 – at least £8,500m at 1979 prices. This represents over a ninth of all public expenditure by central and local government, and around five per cent of the whole national product.[1] To put it in scale picturesquely, the actual money being spent on the NHS each week, if laid end to end in £1 notes, would reach from London to Bangkok and back. We are dealing with very large sums of money, constantly increasing, and not just with statistics in thousands of millions of pounds, or with mere abstract percentages.

The Growth of Expenditure

Figure 1.2 in Chapter 1 showed the scale and trend of NHS expenditure since it began, and its rise from something over three per cent of GDP to four per cent by 1970, and up to five per cent in 1974. Expenditure on health services is agreed by the Cabinet in its decisions on public expenditure. The total of public expenditure includes not only the cost of purchases and labour – 'goods and services' to the economist – but also social security and other transfers. This total is an important figure for public financial policy, and shows what has to be paid for, mainly by taxes, rates and National Insurance contributions. (But the reader should *not* subtract public expenditure from the GDP in order to deduce private expenditure – this (broadly) comes from subtracting from GDP the public expenditure on goods and services, thus leaving aside all transfers from one person to another via the Government.)

Expenditure on the NHS is about one-fifth of public expenditure on 'goods and services.' (i.e. including all labour costs but excluding transfers). Figure 7.1 also gives the trends of these two aggregates of public expenditure. Note that this is not the total expenditure of the 'public sector': it does not include the expenditure of nationalised industries – miners' wages and the like.

Fifteen years ago we spent nearly twice as much on defence as on the health service: now we spend more on the health service than on defence. Following a steep rise in the early 1970s, expenditure on the health service has continued to grow in volume terms (taking account

Figure 7.1: Principal Public Expenditure Programmes by Volume —
Excluding Relative Price Effects

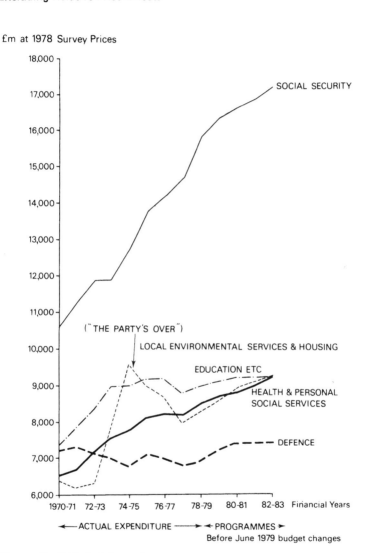

£m at 1978 Survey Prices

Source: See Table 4 of Appendix.

of all inflation) during the recent troubled years when public spending has been restrained. These trends are shown in Figure 7.1. Note that the health line, combined here with personal social services, shows a fairly steady rise, somewhat steeper than for education, and much steeper than for defence: much less steep than the rise in social security payments. Plans for spending on the health services in the January 1979 White Paper[2] allowed for an increase of just under 2 per cent per annum (about the same rate as public expenditure as a whole). The annual percentage changes are shown in Figure 7.2: this shows that the fluctuation on the health programme is less than in the other large programmes.

The Pressures to Spend More

Better Services

There are demands for more staff, more buildings, newer buildings and more equipment. Consider three examples: the growing proportion of elderly people in the population with their increased demands on health care is estimated to require a *growth* of one per cent per annum in NHS expenditure if the Service is merely to *maintain* standards; the timescale for putting right the historic neglect of services for the mentally ill and mentally handicapped was put in recent White Papers[3] as 25 and 20 years respectively, and even these distant dates may not be met, given current restraints; people die from renal failure who could continue to live if there were enough money to provide and run more kidney machines.

For the NHS in the whole of the United Kingdom the current rate of growth (of two per cent per annum) means about an extra £170m a year — averaging less than £2m for each Area Health Authority or the equivalent. We can set this figure alongside estimates of the costs of certain developments: a new District General Hospital costs, say, £25m; a modest reconstruction of old accommodation may cost £100,000; a new consultant post together with supporting services may cost an extra £250,000 a year. Even if the whole of a year's increase were to be spent on increases in nursing staff it would only pay for one extra nurse for every 16 at present working. Given indications of the orders of magnitude of the growth money available and the costs of new developments, we can see that two per cent growth per annum will not by itself go far to finance improvements in health services. We consider in later chapters the difficult but vital task of reappraising the services we now provide so that we do use current resources most effectively.

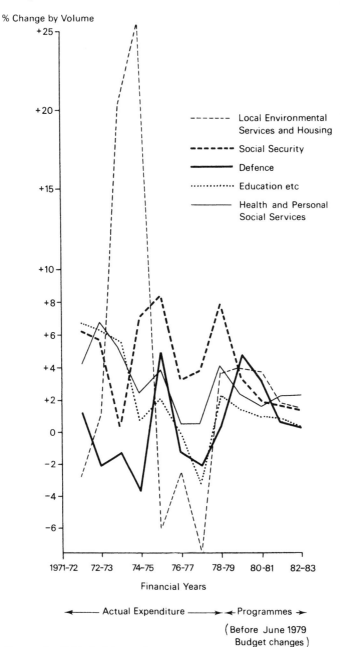

Figure 7.2: Principal Public Expenditure Programmes by Volume — Changes Over Previous Year

% Change by Volume

Local Environmental Services and Housing

Social Security

Defence

Education etc

Health and Personal Social Services

Financial Years

Actual Expenditure ——— Programmes

(Before June 1979 Budget changes)

Source: See Table 4 of Appendix

But there is another source of pressure on NHS resources.

The Pressure for Better Working Conditions

Approaching three-quarters of NHS expenditure is on pay. Reductions in hours worked, or relative increases in pay, can have a massive impact on the cost of the NHS. One way of measuring the effect of giving NHS staff better working conditions is to compare the costs of inputs into the economy (i.e. prices of goods and wages and salaries of workers) with costs of inputs into the NHS. This is illustrated by Figure 7.3. The unbroken line shows how the total NHS costs have moved in relation to national costs. With a labour-intensive concern, when real wages are increasing, relative costs are likely to show an increase. In most years this happened, but particularly in 1974. This followed large pay increases and also the steep rise in building costs in 1972–3. In the following years, there is little rise, or even a fall. The broken line compares costs of NHS consumption (broadly revenue expenditure, nearly three-quarters of which is on staff, even including the family practitioner service) with costs of consumers' expenditure nationally. Very roughly, this gives an indication of the times at which there are big movements in the real remuneration of NHS staff: the effects of pay restraint are seen where this line moves below the unbroken line in 1968 and 1976.

The harsh discipline of bearing the cost of all wage and price increases only partially applies to the NHS. If pay awards allow the real incomes of staff to increase by two per cent per year, this does not normally come out of the planned real growth available to the NHS; if this were the case this would only leave half a per cent growth for improving services for patients. The total health programme is planned on the basis of the 'volume' of expenditure, leaving normal pay and price changes aside. (But within a given financial year, pay settlements made in excess of what is allowed for in the cash limit do cause a squeeze – generally in terms of vacancies having to remain unfilled.) Nevertheless, real increases in pay to those who work in the public sector do have to be financed, and in planning the *total* of public expenditure these and other real increases in pay affect the volume of resources which the nation can afford to devote to the NHS and other public services.

There are considerable pressures to increase the pay of NHS staff. Ancillary workers, for example, have been, and are, among the lowest-paid groups in the community, as indeed are those doing similar work outside the NHS. Their work, though often responsible, is relatively simple and does not demand special qualification and training. In earlier

Figure 7.3: NHS Change in Relative Pay and Prices from Previous Year

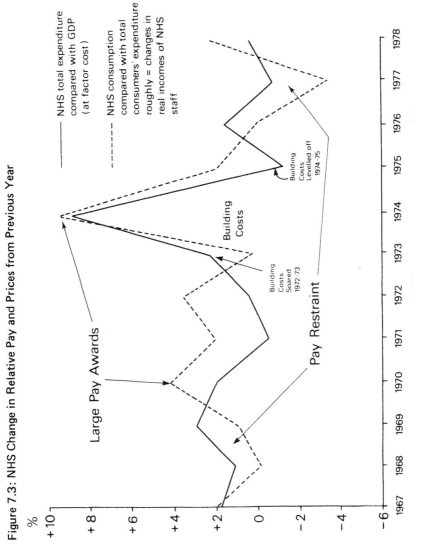

years a rise in pay, relative to many outside jobs, began with the move to equal pay for women, as in other jobs in the public service, and continued with concern over low pay generally. An appropriate comparison is with the national average of female manual earnings: for NHS manual and non-manual ancillary staff the percentage of this average was 99 in 1973, 120 in 1975 and 105 in 1978.[4] The low pay of ancillary workers means that inflation bites immediately on their basic standards of living. In a time of inflation, a major pay award is going to be eroded before the next one comes along. With steep inflation this may be important even during the year between annual pay rounds: one is best off immediately after a pay rise (especially if it has included payment of arrears), and one should *expect* erosion until inflation has been eliminated; living standards have to be planned accordingly. For low-paid groups this is easier said than done: there is little margin over what is generally regarded as basic expenditure.

A second pressure for increases in pay comes from professionals, particularly doctors and nurses. There have been striking changes over the last 50, or even 25 years in the lifestyles of the old professions in this country, except perhaps for successful doctors and lawyers in private practice. The differential compared with manual workers has obviously narrowed greatly. Part of this is no doubt acceptable social change, but many serious and dedicated professionals would feel this had gone too far, and are angry because the main reason for their over-modest pay — mitigated somewhat by the 1979 awards — is that they are in *public* jobs, and not earning from the charges they would otherwise make to their patients. There has also been a change away from a steep progression in pay over a successful doctor's lifetime. The frustration of senior doctors is probably increased by a movement away from a professional attitude by their juniors, reflected in developments such as the charging for overtime, and there is a risk that, with changes in the consultants' contract, this shift in attitude will become more widespread. It is also increased when they are told by their representatives that doctors in, say, Germany and Holland earn much more.[5] British doctors are free to take up jobs in those countries but we have not heard that many do so: the international comparison is therefore rather academic.

We do not examine what the levels of pay should be for these professional jobs — public commissions will be concerned with this in great detail: we are indicating what we see as some of the upward pressures from within the NHS. Pay movements for doctors tend to have wide repercussions inside and outside the public service, though (because numbers are fairly small) the direct cost to the health service is not great. But the pay of nurses is another matter – over 30 per cent of the cost of hospital and community health services (Table 2.3). For reasons we need not go into, they used to be paid what now appear to be unduly low rates. Now, apart from considerations of equity, it is more difficult to recruit nurses. The number of single women wanting jobs in nursing has probably declined; early marriage and family responsibilities, and opportunities for agency nursing and other outside jobs, have made it difficult to maintain full nursing staffs in hospitals. The large pay award made in late 1974 attempted to raise the economic status of nurses in relation to the rest of the community. This increase has been partially eroded by inflation: if again we look at the differential compared with manual workers, nurses in 1973 earned 123 compared with 100 for women's manual work; this rose to 142 in 1975 but fell to 118 in 1978. For male nurses (where manual work includes better-paid jobs than for women) the figures are 78, 104 and 89.[6]

The general problem of pay increases is this. If we can expect a growth of two per cent in national product (more strictly, in real personal disposable income, which allows for the terms of overseas trade), everybody's real income rise, for strong and weak groups, will inevitably average out at two per cent – averaging years in which we overspend and run into massive overseas deficit, and the years when we gradually repay. This is not a large figure, and if some groups actually achieve a higher rise in real terms, others will gain less than two per cent, and indeed may have their real standard of living cut. The vital point is that if everyone gains a large increase in pay, and there is no increase in real product and real disposable income, real incomes as a whole will be no higher – indeed, they may fall because of inflation-any crises and disruption. So a *general* system of large money-wage claims does not increase real incomes, except for the strongest at the expense of the weak. (Later in this chapter we discuss briefly whether deliberate inflation at a time of unemployment may increase real incomes.)

Until industry gets efficient enough to produce and sell more, and there is more national growth to share out, the margin of growth in national income will go on being very narrow. There may be room for *relative* pay increases (and therefore decreases), but when the average growth is so small, the less-favoured groups may have to forgo any increase in real terms, or accept a decrease. Some groups will nevertheless use industrial 'muscle' to get an increase for themselves, and this extends to some groups in the public sector including the NHS. This is all the more likely to happen when pay in the public sector has been held back for some time, and the fight becomes bitter if other groups, perhaps in private employment, are thought to have 'got away with it'. NHS groups have a strong interest in moderation in pay claims generally, since they (especially the lower paid) will feel inflation keenly: and they are unlikely to be in the forefront of those getting big increases in money pay, since the Government both controls their pay and is responsible – to them and to the whole country – for reducing inflation.

We can illustrate the problem by considering the likely effects of a general NHS pay rise of 20 per cent beyond the going rate of wage settlements. This would, for instance, approximately restore the pay of nurses and ancillary workers to the 1975 levels relative to women manual workers. The cost – a broad figure for all staff – would be around £1,300m and be more than seven times the planned real growth of the NHS. Unless such an award had won wide consent within society at large there would be demands for higher wages elsewhere, which would probably erode the real worth of the increase, and/or for a reduction in the volume of NHS resources, which means fewer staff. We conclude that pay will continue to be a difficult and painful subject and that only those NHS groups with a thoroughly convincing case can expect other workers (whose taxes pay for the NHS) to be receptive to claims to move up the relative pay ladder, or to retrieve lost positions; this may be an additional reason why the Government is unwilling to see substantial NHS pay rises.

Allocating More Expenditure to the NHS

The immediate pressures to spend more on the NHS have to be considered by the Cabinet in making their decisions on public expenditure. With a new Conservative Government the emphasis is at present strongly on reductions in total public expenditure, not on increases. The NHS has been fortunate in escaping cuts in the June 1979 Budget, and in maintaining its two per cent increase (in real terms). In a more normal year, with a Government of either the left or the right, the discussion would be the culmination of the thorough Public Expenditure Survey described in Chapter 4. To illustrate the nature of ministerial discussion and decisions on the programmes for health and for all other purposes, we may consider a year when there is general pressure for increases, but when the total of the proposed increases has to be cut down.

The Secretary of State for Social Services will be, let us suppose, trying to win Cabinet approval for an extra two per cent in growth of

NHS expenditure – a modest enough sum, as we have indicated. We can imagine ourselves on an autumn morning in the Cabinet room around the long table trying to decide, within a total which we agreed back in the summer, how public expenditure is going to be allocated. Or rather, since that is far too big a job to do all at once, we are having to decide between the cases put by Cabinet Ministers in charge of, say Health, Housing, Education and Defence, and we can suppose that by the time the Cabinet meets the issues are as follows:

(i) The proposed programmes come to £1,000m more than the total which we set in the summer for the year we are considering – perhaps the second year ahead. (In practice this is a pretty modest excess.)

(ii) The health programme includes limited improvements (four per cent growth instead of two per cent) including one additional large hospital to be built over the next few years, several small units for geriatric and mentally handicapped patients, a further increase in kidney machines and a small increase in medical and nursing staff in order to reduce surgical waiting lists.

(iii) The housing programme also aims to reduce waiting lists for homes, and to make a stronger attack on the conversion of large old existing property, in order to relieve acute deprivation in 'inner city' areas. In place of two per cent in last year's agreed programmes they propose six per cent, an extra £250m. The Housing Secretary says that this appears a rather sharp increase, but that bad housing is one of the causes of lawlessness and vandalism, and an efficient and economical advance will pay dividends.

(iv) The education programme, where children of compulsory school age are declining by over three per cent a year, shows little change in expenditure from year to year. The Education Secretary says that this at least allows a faster reduction in the pupil-teacher ratio, the replacement of more old schools, the payment of maintenance grants to 16 to 18-year-olds continuing at school, and the avoidance of a further increase in the charge for school meals. He says that all this is far less than teachers and parents demand, and that he had not been able to propose increases in university or scientific grants.

(v) The Defence Secretary points out the reductions in recent years in the defence programme, says that the amounts proposed are insuffcient to meet our NATO commitments and that morale is already suffering despite pay increases, and that there is a shortage of skilled men. The Government, he says, has fought an election on the basis of a strong defence programme, and this must be honoured.

These arguments are backed up by some forceful and impassioned speaking by people who care deeply about the particular job they are responsible for. And they are put into focus against the background of the PESC Report (see Chapter 4 above), and later papers by Treasury and spending ministers, which describe in more detail the costs and standards which these decisions would affect. What do you say in that Cabinet room, given that you are not one of the ministers principally affected? You have the painful duty of choosing (let us say) three out of the four programmes for cuts of £300-400m each, and you know that you (as a member of the Government) will have to defend those decisions to the public, and that certain of your colleagues will have to stand up in the House and defend specific changes – even if they are only the deferment of hoped-for improvements.

You have to weigh up, say, £300m worth of marginal measures, as described, for health and for each of the other programmes. You may feel that there ought to be some common measuring-rod which helps you in this – a utilitarian calculus, perhaps, which mobilises the work on measuring health output and that of other public programmes, all seen in the light of your declared policies. But there is no such calculus, and will not be for many years. And whether there is a calculus or not, in some way or other it is you who has to make choices, on behalf of the people who will gain or suffer, between better hospital units for old people, better schools for, say three to five-year-olds, the provision of tolerable housing for down-and-out families, and a noticeable change in the efficiency of the armed forces. This is the point at which either statemanship or political power shows up – and which tests the quality of the chairman, the Prime Minister. It is what you are really elected to Parliament to do, though you are of course now doing it with full responsibility as part of the Government and not in a backbench parliamentary group.

A decision *is* taken: we labour the process of deciding because it shows clearly the sort of costs, and the wide range of the costs, which are attached to a proposal to spend more on health, even on the modest scale described. It is useful to know something of what is in the mind of the Secretary of State when he has to consider what proposals, desired by the health service itself, he will put forward to his colleagues and to the Treasury. Problems within the management of health expenditure also involve this kind of choice: those who deal with patients rather than with money must realise the painful duties which authorities and officers have to face, and must see as much as possible of the nature of the choice so that the decision, once taken, makes some sense to them – even if they do not get exactly what they would have liked.

The Costs of Increasing the Total of Public Expenditure

We have been following the Cabinet's discussions about the allocation of a total which they had already determined after full consideration. The sacrifices which various services must make if other services are to be maintained intact, or developed, have become clear, and decisions have now been taken. These reflect the relative values that ministers collectively have put, for good or bad reasons, on the marginal shifts in the standard of the several services which they have singled out for their final deliberations. We assume that the figure for total public expenditure has held: but now let us move forward 6–8 months to the next decision of this total. What are the arguments for and against a sizable increase – say ten per cent – in two years' time? This idea would be against the policy of the present Conservative Government (and indeed the Labour Government), but we feel that many people interested in social policy – better services, less unemployment, less inequality – do not see why expenditure has to be limited to anything near the present levels, let alone be cut. Nor do some economists who are particularly concerned with reducing unemployment. Let us consider the substance of the argument, as an armchair exercise.

A ten per cent increase (omitting the increases of about two per cent per annum already programmed) would come to around £8,000m at this year's prices – nearly as much as the whole of the present cost of the NHS. This would meet the special pay increases for NHS, teaching and other local authority staff, and allow some modest improvements in a range of services, without giving by any means all that the various services would like. Looking at the percentage of public expenditure to GDP (at market prices), which is a useful rough indicator of the shape of the allotment of national resources, if we were starting from last year's figure of 42 per cent, this would be increased by a tenth (instead of being cut in the June 1979 Budget). The figure would become some 46 per cent; this is in fact the all-time peak figure reached in 1975–6.[7] That percentage in itself may not matter, though the increase in spending plans would be in itself frighten the markets here and abroad, and might bring an another major financial crisis. Whether there would be good reasons for this fright is a different question, and a little far from the central argument of this book, but the subject is so important and difficult to pin down that it seems worth attempting still from our armchair, an exposition of the possibilities of a substantial increase in total public expenditure in the UK in the next few years. It is a matter which is also exercising other governments and international organisations.[8]

Paid for by Tax

Let us suppose first of all that the Government is considering paying for this £8,000m of expenditure by a big increase in taxes, which is contrived so that it roughly neutralises the addition to demand – that is, that the taxes are designed not only so that the public sector borrowing requirement is unchanged but so that the pressure of demand is unchanged, and therefore (in the first instance) that the growth of national production and the level of unemployment are also unchanged. (Economists will realise that this would be a difficult exercise, but will perhaps allow us this oversimplification at the present stage.)

We now have a new set of options to compare – not only health versus education and the rest, but also each of these (being part of the £8,000m package) against the imposition of sacrifices on those who pay income tax, VAT, duties on drink and tobacco, National Insurance contributions. local rates and the rest. It is simple to make a crude comparison with the yield of various taxes. The picture is something like this:

Table 7.1: General Government – Imaginary Accounts for a Future Year

			£m at 1979–80 prices
Public expenditure	80,000	Income tax	24,000
		Expenditure taxes	20.000
		National Insurance contributions	14,000
		Local rates	8,000
		Other income	6,000
		Borrowing*	8,000
Total	80,000	Total	80,000

* For simplicity, let us take this as the General Government Borrowing Requirement and assume that the rest of the Public Sector Borrowing Requirement (i.e. public corporations' outside borrowing) is in balance.

So as to balance an extra £8,000m one has to find ways of reducing people's real incomes by some combination of taxes, and we have (for the present) assumed that this combination must come to £8,000m. To load these amounts onto income tax or National Insurance contributions would lead to ridiculous results. To illustrate this consider what would be necessary:

(i) £8,000m represents a third of the present £24,000m of income tax. Such an increase means a basic rate of 40 per cent rather than 30 per cent with other rates up in proportion (making some marginal rates very high). This would hardly be acceptable to the large number of people who have to pay substantial income tax and economically there would be even less incentive to earn than at present (one can perhaps assent to this proposition even while remaining somewhat agnostic about some of the arguments put forward on taxation and incentives). But it shows the order of magnitude of the purchasing power which would have to be abstracted *by one method or another* if £8,000m were to be found. A man with two children, earning £77 a week gross (£4,000 p.a.), would pay £16 a week in income tax instead of £12 (June 1979 Budget figures). How would he find that extra £4, especially if he is the only wage-earner in the family, and has commitments to pay rent or mortgage interest, hire purchase and the basic expenditure on housekeeping?

(ii) If the same sum were 'put on the stamp' paid by employers and employees, National Insurance contributions would increase by over half. Again, this just would not work. It would have relatively more effect on the lower-paid workers than increasing income tax. And the increase in the employer's contribution − in other words, the tax on employment − is not painless for the worker either. Real income after tax has still got to fall (because you want one group to have more in real terms, and there is no extra national product to share out). There would be some fall in profits, but most of the cost would be loaded on to prices. The results would be that people paid more for the same goods − rather as if VAT had been raised. Export demand would fall but imports would become more competitive. And because their home as well as overseas sales fell, manufacturers would cut back production and employment somewhat, and they would try harder to save labour costs, causing a further drop in employment. So the economic balance the Government was trying to hold would be disturbed by both price inflation and by additional unemployment and depression of demand for home products.

If the extra revenue were to come from VAT (at present £5,000m but rising to £9,000m by 1980−1), taxes on drink (£3,000m), or petrol and oil (£2,000m nearly), enormous proportionate increases would be needed, on top of the steep increases of June 1979. Home production and employment would in some of these cases again be affected, and the necessary drop in real income would mainly come from price inflation arising from the higher indirect taxes that had been imposed.

How far any of these extra impositions would be acceptable depends on people's political attitudes, their expectations as consumers, and on the level of after-tax income that we are starting from. Taking these in turn, if people not only said, 'We must have a better health service', or 'They ought to pay nurses (etc.) better', but also said, 'We accept that taxes will have to go up to pay for what we think ought to be done: and we will be satisfied with lower real take-home pay as a result', it might well be possible to expand public expenditure and to provide better services and more pay for those in special need. There would not be consequential wage increases to make up for the drop in real pay, nor the consequences for price inflation, unemployment and industrial disruption. But we have no such consensus in this country – perhaps because people expect higher spending to be financed, some-how, painlessly, rather than by responsible decision to sacrifice one's private expenditure.

Expectations of high and growing real income, fed over many years by unrealistic plans and promises, mean that people get committed to spend, and cannot face the idea of additional taxation even for a purpose they thoroughly approve of. Real income and expenditure have kept up in crisis years (even in 1974, after the oil price quintupled) but then had to fall sharply to 1977: they rose again in 1978, although production remained low. People respond to being told that there is a crisis, and that belts must be tightened, even for a couple of years: but this is different from cold-bloodedly deciding to pay more for real public services. (Perhaps a lot of people really do think that it is 'the Government', or 'the council', that should be paying, not 'us'.)

Why Not Borrow More?

We have assumed that for our future year, public expenditure exceeds revenue by £8,000m, which is the amount, therefore, of the Public Sector Borrowing Requirement (PSBR), *before* there is any question of spending another £8,000m. How will this money be raised?

In recent years governments have borrowed substantial sums at long term – £5,500m in 1977 and £1,300m in National Savings. This avoids the directly inflationary short-term borrowing from the banks, but it does mean that long-term interest rates are driven up and (indirectly through the exchange rate) that our products become less competitive overseas. To borrow vastly greater sums is contrary to the policy of Labour and Conservative Governments: but it would in any case not be possible – the public would not want to buy so much Government stock. The alternative is large-scale bank finance. Without going into technical detail, this means great pressure for bank lending and a public spending spree of a kind which we have seen in the past, and which has led back to financial crisis.

The restriction of public borrowing to manageable sums is tiresome for the management of economic policy, and even more so for social policy. But this does not mean it can be abandoned without even worse damage, acting through prices, competitiveness and financial crises, on real incomes and on jobs.

Financed by an Alternative Economic Strategy

Some economists and politicians have proposed an 'alternative strategy' which takes various forms but involves the growth of the British ecnomy with protection from overseas competition. Growth would be stimulated by public expenditure, partly on social services but including large amounts of public investment designed to modernise industry and eventually bring it to the stage where it could again compete internationally, at a higher level of efficiency. (This policy would be anathema to the present Government, but if unemployment and low growth are not mastered by their policies, pressures for alternatives will become very strong.)

We consider that those interested in more resources for the health service would be unwise to pin hopes on this strategy. We think the key points are that the industries which have shown weakness would not, in these very restricted circumstances, respond strongly enough to make the breakthrough into higher efficiency which is assumed, and that the experiment could mean shortages and higher costs for some years, great unrest among consumers and some workers at least, and the early reversal of policies for higher social expenditure in the face of acute and prolonged financial crisis. Permanent damage could have been done, and we should still have to find the right industrial and economic solutions.

Our conclusion, sadly, is that the alternative strategy 'will not wash' in the UK, though in other countries it might if their industrial response were strong and swift. So there is no way out there for the NHS – indeed, allocations would inevitably suffer as the real national product fell below its strategic targets.

Expenditure on Health Services as a Proportion of Gross Domestic Product

International Comparisons[9]

Figure 7.4 shows the figures for certain countries in the mid-1970s and in the early 1960s. Expenditure on health is shown in total, and also the public element of this; in some countries there is much more private expenditure on health than in the UK, though the proportion of private to public is tending to decline, sometimes rapidly.

The UK appears fairly low in the chart of these developed and wealthy countries. First, however, it is important to remember that some countries' figures are swollen by the very high earnings of their doctors and others, by the administrative costs of collecting charges (financing through the tax system is highly efficient), and by tendencies to indulge in, or to sell, health treatment (as distinct from the treatment of definite illness and accident) – e.g. Germany and the USA. No doubt a very profitable health industry creates its own demand (health farms, convalescent homes) which it would not necessarily be sensible to encourage. It can, however, be argued that if we were as much concerned with health as other countries we would spend a higher proportion of income on public (or on total) health services. There is something in this, but it is important to remember that the real income per head of several of the other countries is around twice that of the UK, and that the standard of living is higher, even though not always twice as high.

We can explore the significance of this difference by a broad schematic comparison of the UK with a country of twice its real income – 'Plutopia'; it also applies as between the UK and a poorer country (and most countries have far less than half the UK's income). We have dodged the problem that costs of living may be out of line with exchange rates, by not naming the other country.

If we in the UK are thinking of increasing our five per cent on health to, say, eight per cent, disposable income falls from 70 to 67; a similar move in Plutopia means a fall from 140 to 134. The big question is: what does the fall of three mean for the person living in the UK, and what does six mean for the Plutopian? Clearly, the importance for each depends on what cushion he has – on what he has left to spend, or to save. For the Briton, a certain tax increase may mean that he cannot afford to run his car. For the Plutopian, he cannot afford a second car. In the still poorer country, it means that his family does not have enough to eat. Which is the harder to bear? We suggest that because

Figure 7.4: Health Expenditure — International
Comparisons. Percentage of Trend GDP for
Selected Countries of OECD

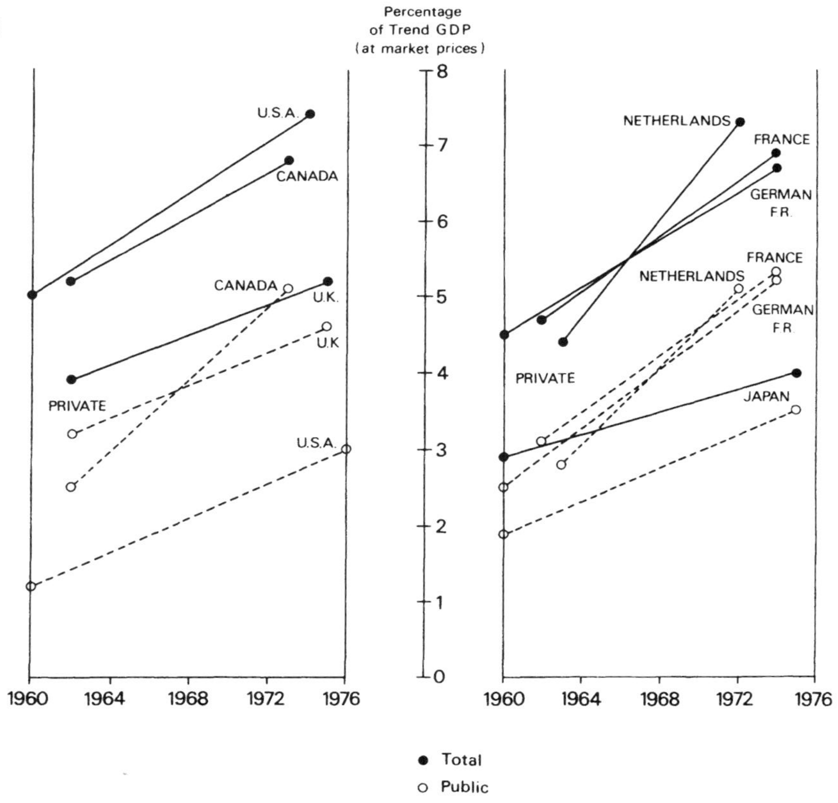

Source: See notes in Statistical Appendix

of the differences in real incomes between different countries there are no simple conclusions to be drawn about the proportion of GDP that ought to be spent on health care. Indeed, one could argue that it is to be expected that poorer countries cannot afford to spend the same proportion of GDP on health services as rich countries choose to do. Yet they may need *more* in the way of basic health services, not less:

Table 7.2: The UK and Plutopia

	UK	Plutopia
GDP/head	100	200
Used by Government etc. for		
Health (5%)	−5	−10
Other services	−25	−50
Disposable income	70	140
Saved	−10	−20
Spent	60	120

this means that they may decide to increase the proportion of GDP going to health, but at great relative cost to their citizens. But the latter may indeed put a high value on health services, as a matter of life and death to them personally. The UK public may not take this view.

Comparisons Within the UK

It is worth considering further the simplistic argument that expenditure on health services should be related to GDP, by a comparison within the UK:

Table 2.3: NHS Expenditure Related to GDP Within the UK

	GP/head*	NHS expenditure— percentage of GDP in each country
England	1,958	4.9
Wales	1,740	5.6
Scotland	1,876	6.1
Northern Ireland	1,506	7.7
UK	1,928	5.1

*From data in *Economic Trends* (November 1978), p. 84.

Unlike the preceding international comparisons, it is clear that the percentage within the UK is higher in the countries with lower GDP. Has the English taxpayer gone too far in paying for higher proportionate health expenditure in the three other countries? If one could produce a similar table for English Regions, would it be argued that the English *percentage* should be kept constant for the regions with lower incomes − for instance, that East Anglia, with under £1,800 per head *needs* less health expenditure than Greater London, with nearly £2,400 a head? If so, the RAWP Report will have to be rewritten! In fact, there is growing emphasis on the need for health expenditure exactly where there is most poverty and deprivation, in parallel with the point we have just made about poor overseas countries. Within the UK this is financed by the whole body of taxpayers, not by those in the area in question. We pursue this point in Chapter 8.

We conclude that comparisons with GDP may have some economic interest, but hardly bear on internal social and financial decisions on health care and expenditure.

Notes

1. One can measure the national product either at market prices or at 'factor cost' − that is, what the employees, suppliers and investors are paid for the product. The difference is substantial because market prices include indirect taxes, which in recent years have added one-ninth to the total price of the product; this will increase with the higher rate of VAT. And it can be measured either as Gross Domestic Product or as Gross National Product, which includes net investment income from abroad. At present this makes little proportionate difference for the UK, but it may for very rich or very poor countries. There are good arguments for using GNP (since the rich countries have extra money which they can apply to health expenditure or to some other purpose whereas the poor countries can sensibly regard their borrowing charges as a deduction from income which they are free to apply). On the other hand GDP is slightly more convenient to apply − it looks at the use of the nation's current product only, splitting this between various uses; and it is used (at market prices) by OECD in their comparative studies and in the UK Public Expenditure White Paper. Various other authors use different measures, sometimes inexplicitly, and the resulting differences in percentage are confusing.* It is also possible to compare NHS expenditure, excluding capital consumption, with Net National Product.

---

* As we go to press we note that the Royal Commission (p. 22 and p. 431 of Cmnd 7615) use GDP at factor cost, and the NHS percentage of GDP is thus higher than in Table 1 of our Appendix. But they implicitly use GDP at market prices in quoting OECD figures on p. 23; the difference is about −0.6 per cent of GDP.

2. *The Government's Expenditure Plans, 1979–80 to 1982–83,* Cmmd 7439 (HMSO, London, 1979).

3. *Better Services for the Mentally Ill,* Cmnd 6233 (HMSO, London, 1975). and *Better Services for the Mentally Handicapped,* Cmnd 4683 (HMSO, London, 1971).

4. *Official Report*, 23 February 1979, cols. 353–6.

5. British Medical Association, *'Report of the New Charter Working Group'*, February 1979.

6. *Financial Times,* 31 January 1979, quoting Treasury figures.

7. 46½ per cent – see *The Government's Expenditure Plans, 1979–80 to 1982–83,* Table 3.

8. *Studies in Economic Growth,* no. 6 (OECD, Paris, 1978).

9. Ibid., no. 5 (OECD, Paris, 1977).

8 ALLOCATING RESOURCES EQUITABLY

The centenary year of Lewis Carroll's publication of a report of a multi-disciplinary team's search for the elusive (and little understood) Snark[1] was celebrated by the publication of the report of the multidisciplinary Resource Allocation Working Party (RAWP) of the DHSS[2]. The RAWP was hunting for a method of achieving the elusive (and little understood) goal of equity in the provision of health care. The report emphasised the elusive nature of this goal by its swingeing criticism of methods used since the inception of the NHS (which it said reflected the inertia of history rather than the need for health care). The RAWP was convinced that past methods were wrong. It was convinced that the methods it had itself proposed in 1975 for measuring morbidity and catering for the extra costs of teaching hospitals were wrong. Finally it was convinced that the methods and principles it proposed in 1976 were not to be challenged in any fundamental way. This conviction is stated thrice[3] in the face of recognised weaknesses in the data being used and the need for research into the factors on which resource allocation decisions ought to be based.

> Just the place for a Snark! I have said it twice:
> That alone should encourage the crew.
> Just the place for a Snark! I have said it thrice:
> What I tell you three times is true.[4]

The Snark turned out to be a Boojum — an end feared by the hunting party. Many already fear the consequences of continuing to follow the RAWP methods in resource allocation.

The Effects of Current Policies

The Change from Incrementalism

The Secretary of State announced in 1976 that he would be broadly following the RAWP principles in making revenue allocations to regions and would be introducing a system over the next few years that followed those principles in making regional capital allocations. The RAWP was particularly critical of the 'incremental' nature of past methods, which tended to allocate future revenue in proportion to past allocations.

137

Table 8.1 gives the forward planning assumptions given by the DHSS to regions for planning purposes for 1978–9 and 1979–80.[5] The table compares the stated allocations for 1979–80 with what this would have been on an incremental basis – i.e. each region receiving the same national growth rate from its 1978–9 allocation.

Table 8.1: A Comparison of Stated Allocations with Incremental Allocations to RHAs for 1978–9 and 1979–80

RHA	1978–9 (1)	1979–80 Actual (2)	1979–80 Incremental (3)	Difference (2) – (3) £m
Northern	249.9	255.1	252.6	2.5
Yorkshire	283.7	287.2	286.8	0.4
Trent	333.6	340.9	337.2	3.7
E.Anglia	138.4	140.9	140.4	0.5
N.W.Thames	342.4	342.8	346.2	−3.4
N.E.Thames	375.0	375.3	379.1	−3.8
S.E.Thames	353.7	354.1	357.6	−3.5
S.W.Thames	275.2	275.6	278.2	−2.6
Wessex	202.2	205.8	204.4	1.4
Oxford	163.4	163.6	165.2	−1.6
S.Western	246.6	250.1	249.3	0.8
W.Midlands	389.2	395.3	393.5	1.8
Mersey	214.3	216.3	216.7	−0.4
N.Western	344.1	351.6	347.9	3.7
Total	3,911.7	3,954.6		

Source: Department of Health and Social Security, *Health and Personal Social Services in England, DHSS Planning Guidelines for 1978–79*, Health Circular HC(78) 12.

The effects of current policies in the immediate future are:

(i) No region has its actual allocation cut.

(ii) The Thames regions, Oxford and Mersey all receive less than they would have done incrementally. All other regions receive more.

(iii) The effects of redistribution are most marked for (a) the Thames and Oxford regions; and (b) N.Western, Trent and Northern regions. The incremental growth forgone by the former finances the greater-than-incremental growth received by the latter.

The Change from Equalisation of Regional Hospital Boards

It is, however, wrong to characterise DHSS policy since 1970 as one of incrementalism: from 1971–2 movements were made towards equalisation amongst Regional Hospital Boards (RHBs). This is not mentioned by the RAWP Report. Table 8.2 gives the different growth rates for each region for the actual allocations made in taking account of the 1970 formula and the RAWP 1976 formula. The later figures are smaller because of the lower growth of the NHS as a whole. But there are marked differences in the relative shares of the growth money.

Table 8.2: A Comparison of Revenue Growth of Regions — The First-year Change as Applied following the 1970 Formula and the RAWP 1976 Formula

Region	1970 formula first-year change as applied 1971—2	RAWP 1976 formula first-year change as applied 1977—8
	Percentage	Percentage
N.Western	6.4	3.2
Trent	5.4	2.9
Northern	3.8	2.9
Wessex	3.7	1.8
W.Midlands	4.5	1.8
E.Anglia	7.4	1.6
S.Western	3.8	1.4
Yorkshire	4.0	1.3
Mersey	2.6	1.1
S.W.Thames	3.8	0.4
Oxford	5.2	0.4
S.E.Thames	3.5	0.3
N.E.Thames	2.6	0.3
N.W.Thames	4.6	0.2

Source: M.J. Buxton and R.E. Klein, *Allocating Health Resources. A Commentary on the Report of the Resource Allocation Working Party* (HMSO, London, 1978), p. 24.

The above figures do not take account of boundary changes, nor, for comparability, do they include allocations for teaching. Even allowing for discrepancies arising from the former omission, there clearly has been a marked shift in the implementation of DHSS policy following the principles of the different formulae. Consider, for instance, the treatment of (i) Trent and Northern; and (ii) Oxford, S.E.Thames, S.W.Thames and N.W.Thames. For 1977—8 the former regions have two of the highest growth rates and the latter the lowest. For 1971—2 the growth rates of Trent and Oxford are similar. Even more striking is the contrast between the Northern and the three Thames regions: for 1971—2 the Northern region received a *lower* growth rate than N.W.

Thames, the same rate as S.W.Thames, and a similar (but slightly lower) rate as S.E.Thames.

There are two other important differences between the policy of 1971–2 and 1977–8. First, until 1974, undergraduate and postgraduate teaching hospitals were financed directly by the DHSS. They were therefore excluded from policies in moving towards equity between RHBs. After 1974, the undergraduate teaching hospitals were brought under RHAs and are included in current policies of redistribution. Second, the equalisation policy introduced in 1971–2 applied to regions only, but the RAWP was asked to produce methods that additionally could be used subregionally. Regions and areas are expected to make judicious use of the RAWP targets in making their allocations to areas and districts. Therefore, in judging the fundamental principles of the RAWP, in terms of a change from the inadequate methods of the past, we shall pay particular attention to how they apply to teaching hospitals and to the making of allocations subregionally.

The Equity Being Sought by the RAWP Principles

The ideal aspired to at the inception of the NHS was equity of access to health care by removing barriers to treatment. The RAWP definition of equity is a relative claim on those resources made available to the NHS in England. Since those resources will not meet current demands for health care, only part of that ideal is now being pursued. And it necessarily follows that people who need and/or demand health care will, in some cases, be denied access to it. The RAWP did not consider rationing in these terms because it specifically excluded from its remit how allocations of money should be used in provision of services. This facilitated the task of the working party, but Health Authorities have still to make these difficult decisions, and the RAWP methods cannot help them do so. (We discuss in the following chapter how this can be done through the planning system.) The RAWP methods are not restricted to remedying geographical discrepancies in service development. In practice the restraint on the well-endowed Thames regions falls most heavily on the London (undergraduate) teaching hospitals. These institutions are of national importance, and the cuts imposed on them cannot be seen purely as a reduction of relative overprovision for their local population. Cuts affect the provision of rare specialties (in some cases for the whole country), the training of over half the medical students in England, and medical research.

These two points raise doubts about the value of the RAWP principles in their formulation of equity beyond that pursued by the DHSS after 1970. In the extended review that follows, we amplify the concerns illustrated by these points. We consider how useful the targets derived from the RAWP methods are in guiding regions and areas in making their respective allocations to areas and districts. We discuss how the policies for the development of undergraduate teaching hospitals in London are illuminated by using the RAWP targets and the estimate of the Service Increment for Teaching; and how the problems of London can be resolved by the London authorities: the RAWP Report was convinced that the authorities would be able to determine the appropriate pace of change. The RAWP principles and methods are criticised in the next three main sections. First, there are the principles that arose from the terms of reference: the use of one method to guide allocation at each administrative level and the exclusion of general practice and local authority services from the assessment of needs for health care to be provided by Health Authorities. Second, there is the principle that equity is primarily determined by resident population. Third, there is the methodological principle that methods of resource allocation can be developed independently of how resources are to be deployed. We follow this review of the principles with a general appraisal of the methods that follow in using these principles in resource allocation.

The Principles of the Terms of Reference

The terms of reference were:

> To review the arrangements for distributing NHS capital and revenue to RHAs, AHAs, and Districts respectively with a view to establishing a method of securing, as soon as practicable, a pattern of distribution responsive objectively, equitably and efficiently to relative need and to make recommendations.[6]

A Universal Method for Calculating Targets

The RAWP interpreted these terms of reference as requiring a universal method applicable to RHAs, AHAs and Health Districts. This interpretation, completed with the RAWP statement that resource *deployment* was outside its remit,[7] means that the methods chosen become increasingly inapplicable as the administrative units to which they relate become smaller. A corollary was that the RAWP 'had perforce to consider only those criteria, the supporting statistical data for which are readily available and reliable at all three levels of disaggregation required'.[8] This constraint resulted in three highly contentious uses of data: the estimate of the Service Increment For Teaching; the use of Standardised Mortality Ratios as a surrogate measure of morbidity; and the whole approach to the derivation of capital targets.

The Exclusion of General Practice and Local Authority Services

The RAWP recognised the effect of local authority services on the need for health care. The RAWP argued that because these lie within other social programmes they were not equipped to deal with these issues and that it would be wrong to correct for deficiencies in these services in any permanent way in making allocations for health care. But they recognised that in the short term such deficiencies would impose an added burden on Health Authorities which would have to be taken into account in phasing allocations to move towards the RAWP criteria of equity. General practitioner services are part of the health programme but were excluded in the terms of reference. They are currently funded separately from Health Authorities. The RAWP view was that 'It is, to say the least, credible that the effect of the separate funding arrangements and the lack of a common need base may well lead to diverse and possibly incompatible planning decisions.'[9] And it recommended a review of the interaction between the services, in terms of the resource effects.

One of the principles of the reorganised NHS is to encourage the co-ordination of services provided by local government, hospitals and general practice. Yet the basis of funding each of these services remains distinct. The introduction of resources earmarked for projects jointly financed by Health Authorities and local authorities does not remove the force of this criticism. The very limited resources made available are meant as a catalyst for joint action. This innovation is official recognition of the failure of reorganisation to overcome one of the weaknesses of the NHS prior to 1974. (This may, however, also be due to financial restraint, each type of authority being reluctant to develop services that might be provided by the other.)

The Principle of Resident Population

The Use of Resident Population in the Calculation of Targets

Fundamental to the calculation of a target is the resident population of the authority (or district). In the calculation of revenue targets some account is taken of patients receiving treatment by a different authority (or district) from that in which they live. But the general principle in the calculation of capital targets is that these flows should cease and the targets be dominated by the residential population. Although the RAWP approach is intended to aid the phasing of resource allocation to achieve equity in the medium to long term, the methods themselves provide no basis for a phased movement that balances capital and revenue. The only methods that can do so subregionally are those that consider how resources are to be deployed (a point we pursue later).

One of the report's weaknesses is its focus on allocations to regions rather than to areas and districts also. The report mentions the problem of allocations within regions, but does not touch on what we consider to be a critical point in determining capital and revenue development – the desirable degree of self-sufficiency of a subordinate authority or district. We were often told by NHS staff that district self-sufficiency was departmental policy – a finding that was responded to by DHSS staff with dismay. Since the report, the DHSS has come out clearly against the mistaken interpretation of their policy as district or area self-sufficiency. In clarifying this position on 27 September 1977 the then Secretary of State mentioned that some had wrongly interpreted the RAWP Report as endorsing local self-sufficiency.

Accounting for Day and Out-Patient Services

No allowance is made in RAWP for cross-boundary flows for day and out-patient services, because of the lack of data. The RAWP Report noted: 'Outpatients represent almost as large a proportion of NHS expenditure as all psychiatric patients, yet virtually nothing is known about their characteristics and movements.'[10] In promoting efficient use of resources the department encourage hospitals where possible to provide treatment that does not involve patients staying in hospital. Some minor surgery, for instance, can be performed during a day and the patient be discharged without being admitted as an in-patient. If the patient is from ouside the administrative boundary of the unit providing treatment, no credit is gained for its RAWP target for such efficient practice.

Accounting for In-Patient Services

The RAWP target does include an allowance for cross-boundary flow of in-patients, but methods are currently handicapped by inadequacies in data of costs and of patients. Cross-boundary flows may be of two kinds: it may be more convenient for a patient who lives in one authority to receive treatment in another, or a district may be responsible for an area, region or even national specialty. The RAWP methods use the average costs of treatment to compensate for both kinds of cross-boundary flow. This is unlikely to be appropriate. If we consider the costs of various types of treatment, we may expect many of them to cluster together — these will be the common kinds of treatment being offered. There is likely, however, to be a significant proportion of much more expensive kinds of treatment within each of the specialties for which average costs are used to account for cross-boundary flow. These treatments are unlikely to be generally available and will tend to be offered by certain hospitals for patients coming from a very wide area, for example, regional and national specialties. Although we do not know the distribution of these costs, because the data are not easily determined by current NHS information systems, we can deduce a likely pattern given that cases are believed to form this sort of double group:

Figure 8.1: Distribution of Cost of Treatment

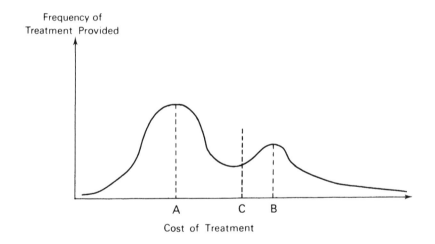

This distribution is really the combination of two different distributions: costs that cluster around the mode at A would correspond to treatments provided at District General Hospitals; those that cluster around B would correspond to the more expensive national and regional specialties. The average cost of the specialty as a whole would lie between A and B, at C. One of the characteristics of distributions of this nature is that C would be significantly greater than most of the costs of treatment provided at District General Hospitals (and because of skewness may be nearer to B than to A). This means that using average costs of treatment not only fails fully to compensate regional and national specialties – a point commonly recognised – but it also over-compensates for the normal treatments given by hospitals to patients from outside their administrative boundaries.

A second problem arising from this distribution is that the method used to estimate the average costs is the statistical technique of regression analysis. One of the assumptions of regression analysis is that the variables being estimated should be 'normally distributed'. The estimates may be robust to violations of this assumption but, since we do not know how skew these actual distributions are we cannot know how much in error are the estimates arising from this assumption. An additional problem with accounting for cross-boundary flow is that the data used on patient treatment are notoriously inaccurate. These data are not always checked, and even where checks are made which discover significant errors, corrective action appears to be exceptional. Currently quite significant sums are allocated to targets based on unreliable data on patients.

Accounting for Regional and National Specialties

The RAWP Report suggested that though improvements in data were desirable, they would be unlikely to call its principles into question. Research is in hand on providing cost data. Whilst these data provide the opportunity for accounting more adequately for allocating resources to hospitals whose expensive specialties serve a wide area, two further difficulties arise.

The DHSS, for instance, cannot merely identify the very high cost of treatment of some national specialties and guarantee to fund cross-boundary flows to these specialties in making its allocation to that region. It may be necessary to set an upper limit in terms of the physical facilities for treatment, in cases where there appears to be need for *national* policy on the use of expensive resources. In some cases the treatment can be shown to be cost-effective in terms of savings made, e.g. from not having to treat, throughout their lives, the babies that would have been born defective. Other cases either give a different result or cannot be assessed in this way, and decisions on resource constraints may mean an explicit limit on treatment that can prevent death (e.g. open-heart surgery).

A second difficulty is that districts which administer regional and national specialties not only currently have less attributed to their RAWP targets than they are likely to be entitled to, but also have a more intensive take-up by their own residents than by those from elsewhere. This is the familiar problem of supply influencing demand. So that even if costs are identified and districts receive full compensation for cross-boundary flow they will still incur extra expense which will not be accounted for by the RAWP methods: it is balanced presumably by extra benefits for their residents — but this means cutting down on services in other specialties. The core of this problem is that in practice access to health care is heavily influenced by proximity to supply;[11] the provision of services in one locality to serve a wide area means that access to these services will be unequal.

Ways of Achieving Equity

The RAWP methods allow financial targets for each administrative unit of the NHS to be calculated. The principle of moving towards these targets is that 'there would eventually be equal opportunity of access to health care for people at equal risk',[12] and that this should be achieved by providing buildings and staff commensurate with targets based on the resident population of each unit. Under current policies equity might be best achieved in this way. But it would seem easier to move patients than relocate existing staff and buildings. Might there not be other ways of moving towards equity which make more efficient use of existing resources? And given the very slow movement that we can expect towards equity with the limited resources available for distribution, might not other ways be more efficacious? Alternatives worthy of investigation include, as suggested by Buxton and Klein,[13] the provision and/or subsidisation of transport, and improvement of information about spare capacity for various kinds of treatment. None of this is straightforward. Those receiving long-stay care ought to be reasonably close (but how close must this be?) to their relatives and friends. But the separation of long-stay from acute care runs counter to attempts to integrate both to avoid the isolation of long-stay institutions. These difficulties do not mean that such policies can be ignored. Their thorough investigation may produce a strategy that does more for the achievement of equity than following the RAWP principles ever will. (This seems to be especially pertinent to the outer areas of the Thames regions which tend to have good connections with the well-endowed inner areas.)

The Methodological Principle of Separating the Allocation and Deployment of Resources

The RAWP Principles and Planning

The RAWP Report emphasised that it was concerned with the allocation of financial resources and not how resources are deployed (i.e. the allocation of money to administrative units, not service developments). This is a useful separation of the DHSS to make because it means that regional plans cannot reasonably be bids for extra resources (although this was not universally realised in the first planning round). Resources are allocated following the RAWP principles, and decisions on how best to use those resources have to be resolved through planning. But even at this level the RAWP Report was aware that there could be a mismatch between the allocations of capital and revenue based on the RAWP targets.[14] Subregionally these problems become more severe. Not only is it wasteful to give a district, say, extra revenue just because it is below its revenue target (if the district cannot redeploy or acquire either the buildings or the staff to make good use of it), but more importantly, decisions on capital are not merely matters of financial equalisation (in the long or the short term) but are about the *kind* of extra resources to be deployed. It is vital to avoid duplicating existing resources, although there is pressure to do so when authorities seek self-sufficiency. What is required are decisions about which cross-boundary flows ought to be maintained and which ought to be eventually eliminated.

Decisions on cross-boundary flow are strategic: they are fundamental to the formulation of the capital programme. They must therefore be resolved by strategic planning. Because this responsibility is vested in both regions and areas, resolution of these issues is not straightforward. The regional strategic plan is intended to draw upon area strategic plans. (This commonly did not happen in the first planning round because area plans arrived too late to be useful to regions.) The regional plan would then be able to draw on the areas' proposals and formulate its policy on cross-boundary flows. But before areas can produce their strategic plans they need resource guidelines from the region. The region can only give such guidelines when it has made decisions on cross-boundary flow. Strategic planning in the NHS therefore includes a process of negotiation over resources. The RAWP targets do provide focal points for those negotiations but they can only be of limited value because the crucial decisions at this level are very much about the kind of services to be developed — matters deliberately excluded from the RAWP approach.

National Priorities and RAWP

In 1976, through the planning system, the DHSS began to promulgate a change in priorities for health care[15] but the RAWP principles are based on past patterns of expenditure. In practice the effect on *targets* of the different priorities revenue is estimated to be quite small (about 0.2 per cent on average).

What is more important is the way RAWP accounts for the mentally ill and the mentally handicapped. The approach is based on an estimate for each region of the number of in-patients it should expect to have in hospitals, based on the national average. If a region has fewer in-patients than this estimate, it is assumed that other regions are treating these patients, and the target is reduced by the estimated cost of treatment. One region estimates that because of this its target was cut by £4m. Now DHSS priorities for the mentally ill and the mentally handicapped are intended to encourage the development of care in the community. But regions which pursue this policy most assiduously will be penalised through RAWP because they will have a lower number of in-patients than would be expected at the rates of the national average. A more general problem arising from the separation of allocation and deployment within the RAWP methods is that there is a potential conflict between moving towards RAWP targets, and DHSS priorities for service developments. Within one region at least, above-target areas have inadequate psychiatric services. Developing these is a national priority but this would push the areas' actual expenditure further in excess of their targets.

Setting RAWP Capital Targets

We have argued that the RAWP approach to capital is seriously flawed because of its inadequate treatment of cross-boundary flow. The methods of determining capital targets are further weakened by the poor data on which they are based. In measuring available capital stock the RAWP faced the difficulty that there was no adequate, up-to-date survey of NHS capital. The most recent relevant data were those of a 1972 Hospital Maintenance Survey which asked RHBs for proportions of floor area in three age categories: pre-1918, 1919–48, 1949–61. This survey had an 80 per cent response rate in which teaching hospitals were under-represented, and no statement is made about the reliability of these data. Other data of doubtful accuracy (SH3) were used to estimate floor area in non-responding hospitals. It was also assumed that the age distribution in non-responding hospitals is the same as in those which did respond. Age of capital stock does not alone indicate its fitness or appropriateness. These also depend on maintenance and location. It was beyond the scope of RAWP to provide measures that took account of these. Instead, depreciation factors were estimated for the three age groups. These were applied to beds on the basis of £24,000 for an acute bed and £12,000 for a non-acute bed. From 1962 the actual capital expenditure in each year was depreciated and added to the value of the pre-1962 stock to give a total valuation.

This approach is based on a succession of heroic assumptions. The overriding impression given by a reading of these sections of the report is of a drive to produce some measure of capital stock in the short time available, however inadequate that measure might be. The only test mentioned of the sensitivity of the outcome of the assumptions made, is that varying the depreciation factors for the three periods of the 1972 survey was found to have no significant effect. But in the critique of the RAWP Report by the Radical Statistics Health Group, an illustration is given of a relatively minor change in depreciation factors which does have a significant impact on the ranking of the different regions.[16]

In the equalisation of capital it is vital to have a good measure of existing stock because the capital investment of the past is many times greater than the new capital available in any year. Table D1 of the RAWP Report[17] shows that in the 1972 survey nearly 65 per cent of English hospital floor area existed in buildings constructed before 1918. For a region making capital allocations to areas it is hard to see how the RAWP approach to valuing this stock gives a measure of its usefulness.

In our report a different approach was recommended from that of the RAWP Report – the method adopted by Wessex RHA, which develops a framework for capital investment by identifying deficiencies in existing stock.[18] This approach relates the framework for capital equalisation to the planning process, and it is through that process that capital allocations will be made subregionally. The DHSS can separate resource allocation from planning, and in making allocations to regions the capital approach they have developed might be appropriate. But it would also seem proper that the NHS should develop a sound valuation of its existing stock so that these regional allocations can be more soundly based.

The London Teaching Hospitals

The principles of RAWP were to identify an earmarked allowance for the extra costs of teaching – the Service Increment For Teaching (SIFT) – which taken together with the elements of a target for a non-teaching district (or area) would produce a target for a teaching district. If the current allocation is considerably in excess of the target, the inferences to be drawn are that this sum ought to be available for service provision, and that the existing allocation perhaps ought to be cut, and the money saved ought to be distributed throughout the regions. We gain an indication of the nature of these excesses by examining the way in which the SIFT was estimated.

The excess costs of teaching hospitals are derived by deducting an estimate of 'service costs' from their actual costs. The estimate of service costs are provided by the '45 Sample Hospital Formula' (used by the department to assess revenue costs of new hospitals). This formula gives cost estimates which are higher than the average running costs of non-teaching hospitals. The excess costs of teaching are divided by the number of students to give this distribution:

Figure 8.2: Distribution of Excess Costs of Teaching

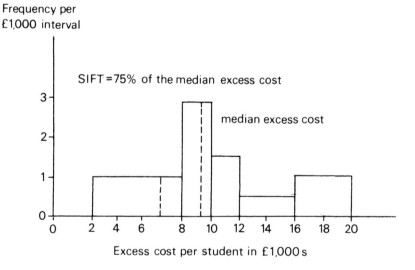

Source: Department of Health and Social Security, *Sharing Resources for Health in England,* Report of the Resource Allocation Working Party (the RAWP Report) (HMSO, London, 1976), p. 49.

This distribution has a rather peculiar shape. The RAWP Report suggests two explanations for the wide spread in these excess costs (with Westminster put at £19,100 and Newcastle at £3,300 per student). Each results from the failure to estimate the costs of services provided other than teaching. The formula used overestimates costs of running a normal hospital and therefore has subtracted too much at the lower end of the range. It would not, however, cover the costs of research and expensive specialties of hospitals at the top end of the range. In the above distribution three measures of central tendency lie within the interval of £8,000–10,000: the mean is at 9.7, the mode at 9.0 and the median at 9.5. The median cost was taken as the starting point. The hospitals in this interval are: Liverpool (£8,000), Guy's (£8,200), Middlesex (£8,700), University College (£9,300) and the London (£9,500). The report pointed out that these hospitals enjoy a reputation for research and provision of regional and national specialties. Neither of these factors ought to have been included in the estimate of the service costs and will therefore have been erroneously included in the estimated costs of teaching. Thus the median cost of £9,500 is over-generous, and the report guesses that 75 per cent of this figure is a reasonable allowance for the excess costs per student (£7,125).

The histogram shows that the majority of teaching hospitals have excess costs greater than that allowed for by the SIFT. Fifteen out of twenty hospitals are in this position – which includes every London teaching hospital and Bristol, Liverpool and Oxford. There are two principles at stake here. The first is the general concept of attempting to separate out the costs of teaching. If teaching cannot be meaningfully disentangled from research and the practice of advanced medicine, these costs cannot properly be identified. Second, the consequences of using the SIFT to guide resource allocation are to squeeze the London teaching hospitals. In terms of the proliferation of specialties it might well seem that cuts in resources going to these hospitals ought to be made. But these cuts have to be decided in terms of what can be best dispensed with and what ought to be preserved. It is hard to see how the SIFT provides a useful guide here. It is supposed to protect the costs of teaching but it may be that these costs could be reduced in London, compared with provincial hospitals, if the teaching hospitals can arrange to share facilities. It excludes the costs of research, which may be of national importance.

The DHSS Strategy of Resource Allocation

The two important differences between current DHSS policies in moving towards equity in resource allocation and policies prior to reorganisation, are that they include teaching hospitals, and that the DHSS is attempting to influence subregional allocations. There are two paradoxes in each of these differences. We begin by highlighting their nature and then explain how they can be understood as rational action in negotiation over resources.

The Paradoxical Treatment of London Teaching Hospitals

The purpose of including undergraduate teaching hospitals within the new RHAs was to make regional planning easier. Away from London this is a sound reason. But it does not make sense in London. In 1956 Anne Godwin, in her note of dissent in the report of the Guillebaud Committee, argued for bringing the teaching hospitals under the RHBs.[19] But she saw special problems with London and advocated that this change be tried first with provincial hospitals and only be applied to London with the benefit of that experience. The 1968 report of the Royal Commission of Medical Education (the Todd Report)[20] recommended bringing all teaching hospitals within the regional structure, but considered that there were too many teaching hospitals north of the Thames to be easily accommodated by two regions, and recommended three regions for this purpose. Those who work in the two North Thames regions of the reorganised NHS would certainly not see the inclusion of teaching hospitals as facilitating their planning.

One deleterious facet of the current structure is that decisions of national importance in the balance between services, teaching and research may be forced upon areas and districts. The DHSS has already had to intervene to stop an AHA cutting back the resources of teaching hospitals in order to provide resources for the development of community services. And the DHSS has established the London Planning Consortium to take a grip on the problems of London. This body is composed of representatives of the London regions and the DHSS (in the chair).

The problems of London are not new. The Todd Report commented that they have been 'obvious enough for many years, and there have been many attempts to solve them. But their roots go deep into history and no solution easily agreeable to all interested parties is likely to be found.'[21] The Todd Report recommended radical changes in terms of reducing the twelve medical schools to six, but the recommendation was not implemented, and in 1978 the Comptroller and Auditor General commented that little progress had been made on the more limited recommendation of rationalisation.[22] These problems are essentially national not regional problems, and RHAs are not best equipped to tackle them. What is peculiar is that up to 1974 the DHSS ought to have been well placed to take the necessary action. Until that time teaching hospitals were funded and administered directly by the DHSS. What is even more surprising is that the movement to regional equity which began in 1971—2 concerned Regional Hospital Boards and omitted teaching hospitals, but from 1976 the adverse effects of moving towards regional equity bore most heavily on teaching hospitals. What has happened since 1974 is that the DHSS has cut undergraduate teaching hospitals off from their direct administrative line, and indirectly imposed a stringent financial policy which (it seems) would have been best implemented with that line still intact. This appears to be a difficult and damaging situation, and a paradoxical way of handling institutions of national importance.

The Paradox of Quantitative Targets

It must be appropriate to seek for some measure of sickness to guide resources to those places with the greatest need for health care. The RAWP's use of Standardised Mortality Ratios (SMRs) has been criticised as a poor measure of morbidity, but since all measures are contentious there is no simple way of resolving this continuing debate. The RAWP Report recognises these difficulties: 'we are conscious of the probability that any allocation method based upon the data available may be open to challenge on grounds which will be difficult to either substantiate or refute'.[23] This consciousness is well judged. What is remarkable is the (first) statement of conviction that follows: 'we are convinced that the data we have used are sufficiently reliable to support the conclusions and methods we propose'.[24]

The problems arise partly from persisting with the use of a quantitative formula when morbidity cannot even be defined. A fundamental step in achieving the level of quantitative measurement ideally required for use in the RAWP calculations is to be able to define the zero of the scale in terms of the absence of the property being measured. Even at the pragmatic level of defining sickness in terms of available, known, effective treatments, it follows that the definition changes as new treatments are discovered. At regional level the crude surrogate of SMRs may suffice, but subregionally these data are subject to considerable instability. Since the RAWP methods assume a linear relationship between SMRs and resource allocation for health care, these variations have a significant impact on subregional targets. The RAWP may be right in their convictions that 'formulae should be the chief determinant of allocations from the DHSS to RHAs'.[25] But to use formulae sub-regionally to guide allocations towards unstable targets based on surrogate estimates appears to be a questionable improvement on methods of the past.

It might have been more appropriate to use SMRs for allocations to regions and seek for some other measure to be used subregionally. But the RAWP considered that they were committed to one method at each administrative level. It was the requirement of a sound national data base, together with the importance of choosing data that were not in-fluenced by supply, that led the RAWP to choose SMRs. Caseloads (used in the RAWP interim report) and waiting lists are influenced by supply, and were rejected on this ground as an indicator of need in the final report. Other indicators discussed but rejected were payment of sickness benefit, self-reported sickness and past *ad hoc* surveys of morbidity. None of these met the criterion of a sound national data base that applied to the whole population. Mortality statistics did meet this criterion. These data had the added attraction that *if* they were good surrogates for morbidity they 'present an opportunity to relate differential morbidity to health care need by reference to con-ditions that no other sources permit'.[26] Allocating resources according to demand is self-defeating because supply fuels demand. Allocating resources according to SMRs is also self-defeating because, as the RAWP recognised, 'the prevalence of many conditions which are among the main causes of mortality is probably not significantly influ-enced by the intervention of health care services'.[27] This observation makes it all the more remarkable that the RAWP proposed a linear relationship between SMRs and resource allocation.

Rational Action in Resource Allocation

There are two paradoxes in DHSS policies on resource allocation. First, the RAWP aimed to improve methods of allocating resources by quanti-fying morbidity — a characteristic that defies definition. Second, the DHSS has subjected the London teaching hospitals to cuts in resources to be implemented by Health Authorities, although a national policy ought to be formulated which is beyond the scope of those authorities. These paradoxes can be understood when we appreciate that the DHSS is involved in negotiation over resources. We commonly try to explain actions in terms of an underlying consensus. When parties are in conflict over resources this consensus has yet to be negotiated. In negotiation the most effective strategies often do not appear to be immediately rational.[28]

Worsening Communications

Common strategies in negotiation are to employ an agent to negotiate, to make threats and then make communication difficult if not impossible.[29] The policies of the DHSS with respect to undergraduate teaching hospitals, since 1974, are open to being seen as the implementation of such a strategy. Direct negotiation was replaced by using RHAs as agents, and the threats were made by introducing revenue targets which are significantly below the current expenditure of most teaching areas.

Communication by Focal Points

In negotiation each party does not know how much to believe of threats that are made. A union negotiator may threaten a strike if his demands are not met, but no one can be certain that he really means his threat or can bring it about. Even the union representative cannot be sure that men who agree to *threaten* a strike will carry out that threat. If an inner London area threatens to make cuts on its teaching districts the districts may threaten to take unpopular action which adversely affects the public. They might, if cuts are imposed, not take such action but seek other economies. The management of the district may not know what is feasible with reduced resources until it is perfectly clear that the district will have to cope with these reductions. In a changed environment of this kind, options which had previously been ruled out as quite impossible are found on reappraisal to turn out to be feasible. Communication in negotiation must lie in the spectrum between perfect communication and none. If we take the extreme assumption of no communication and consider how people can co-ordinate, we gain understanding of the role of focal points in negotiation. Experiments have shown that people can co-ordinate tacitly,[30] i.e. without communication – providing there is conspicuous point on which to focus. If, for example, we are asked to pick a number that we would expect others to select from 0,14,15,16,17 or to choose a place to meet on an island which the map shows has only one house, then we focus the conspicuous features. In negotiations agreement is quite often made similarly. Governments, in attempting to influence wage bargaining, pick on numbers such as £6 per week, 10 per cent or 5 per cent. Round numbers are often seen as rallying points: 10 per cent has, for instance, been picked out as of particular significance in increases in the retail price index and in the mortgage interest rate. Often in negotiations the status quo is a crucial influence and may be seen to determine the outcome. In this respect the incremental allocations of the past in the NHS are typical outcomes of bargaining.

The existence of conspicuous solutions does not remove the scope for bargaining skill but shifts its nature. Skilled negotiators do not concentrate exclusively, or even primarily, around a focal point, but also attempt to structure the negotiation in such a way that the solution which appears to be conspicuous is in their favour. The role of the RAWP targets is to replace existing budgets as conspicuous influences on future allocations.

The Achievements of the RAWP Report

Despite all the criticism that can be made of the RAWP Report, it has registered the massive achievement of changing the basis of resource allocation in the NHS. No longer is last year's budget seen as the factor of overriding importance in allocating next year's money. The RAWP targets, however crude, have the vital impact of causing those authorities with heavy expenditures to justify these, rather than take them as a *prima facie* claim on the lion's share of next year's growth money.

The Limitations of the RAWP Methods

The problem facing authorities is that, while the RAWP principles have overcome the inertia of maintaining the status quo, they provide no basis for a different system. This is because decisions about resource allocation cannot be sensibly separated from decisions about deployment. In particular, the innovatory features of the RAWP approach compared to DHSS policy since 1970 (extending the principle of equity to subregional allocations and undergraduate teaching hospitals) are seriously flawed as a guide to future action. And even at regional level the RAWP Report recognises that the current systems can produce a mismatch between the allocations of capital and revenue. Subregionally the coarseness of the methods and the instability of the targets to changes in population data (which include SMRs) must mean that they can only be of very limited value.

There is, however, a more fundamental matter which was not touched upon by the RAWP Report. This is the problem of facing up to what we mean by rationing in terms of what is to be forgone. If we aim for equal access for all, but if access to all kinds of health care that the community needs cannot be afforded, then what rationing is to be introduced? Until recently the rationing has been in terms of geography. Those with access to London had a privileged access that could not be afforded on a uniform basis throughout the country. The RAWP, by introducing rationing by finance on a geographical basis, necessarily implied that this system, which had persisted for nearly thirty years, was to end.

But there is no guidance as to how authorities are to ration. We argued in Chapter 2 that what is now seen as the disproportionate share of resources allocated to teaching hospitals might be reasonable if one could assume that economic growth would ensure that the treatments provided there would in time become available to the whole country. It was to be expected that the rationing imposed by the RAWP would immediately cause a crisis in London. But again, the RAWP approach provides no means of knowing how to resolve this problem, and the RAWP believed that this could be resolved by the Health Authorities concerned. What is at issue is not merely changing the basis of negotiation between authorities in the NHS, but for the much deeper question of what sort of health service we want. The problems of the London teaching hospitals are at the core of this question.

The Problems of London

The Vice-Chancellor of the University of London has asked a committee under the chairmanship of Lord Flowers to investigate the future of medical education in London and to examine the situation of the London medical and dental schools. It is considering how medical education in London should be reorganised, and the possible phasing-out of one or more medical schools. But the savings from closing a London undergraduate teaching hospital for the NHS as a whole are unlikely to be large. If we presume that the patients will still need to be treated and the students still need to be trained, it is not at all clear that the consequences of a major relocation exercise would save very much – if, indeed, there were any savings at all.

Other less radical changes would be for teaching hospitals to share resources: for example, hospital A would specialise in and teach cardiothoracic surgery, hospital B neurosurgery. This approach does have disadvantages for doctors and students through not having all facilities on the same site. It would also cause problems for some patients since often the different kinds of expensive care are required by the same patient. A second possible rationalisation would be to merge the small preclinical departments of those medical schools which take large numbers of students from Oxford and Cambridge and other places for clinical training.

Again this poses logistic problems, and the savings are unclear and may not be large. One impediment to rationalisation is that in the proposed merging of two undergraduate teaching hospitals (as recommended by the Todd Report[31]) each sees little benefit from the effects of the proposal. But if mergers were considered between undergraduate and postgraduate education, each institution might see advantages. This might mean taking the London undergraduate teaching hospitals outside the regional structure again: this may be the best way of maintaining their high standards under the future constraints on resources.

Under current policies (of not actually cutting revenue to the Thames regions) the costs of maintaining excellence in the inner London areas are the deprivation of the areas in the Thames regions outside central London. In quantitative terms the RAWP gives an estimate of excess residual costs on average of each London teaching hospital of approximately £1.1m (at 1975–6 prices).[32] However, in practice, the discrepancies from using RAWP targets are of a different order of magnitude. One teaching AHA was £20m in excess of its long-term RAWP target. This area has three teaching hospitals and the RAWP Report estimates the excess costs of these hospitals to be less than £3.5m. The reason for this enormous discrepancy between the two methods is that the RAWP Report used the 45 Sample Hospital Formula to estimate the costs of running a general hospital, and the RAWP targets for services are based on a division of resources allocated to the NHS on the RAWP components of resident population and cross-boundary flow. It seems that standards of service throughout the country must therefore be significantly less expensive than the estimates of the 45 Sample Hospital Formula.

The difference between these two estimates is of enormous significance. For instance, one teaching district we visited was aiming to reduce its revenue expenditure by £250,000 each year. Now in terms of the area's excess over its RAWP target (of £20m) these cuts appear to be a minuscule effort. But we were told that within a few years the continuation of such cuts would severely impair either the service or the teaching functions of the hospital. And the RAWP report shows that the estimate of this hospital's excess cost is only £250,000. Therefore, after one year's cut of £250,000, this district would have achieved its baseline service cost (as estimated by the 45 Sample Hospital Formula) including its national allowance for SIFT. It is not therefore surprising that continuing to make cuts would be seen to impair the functions of the hospital: yet much larger cuts have to be made to get to the RAWP target.

The fundamental issue is therefore how far we cut resources going to the London teaching hospitals. It seems that they are being required to go below those of the 45 Sample Hospital Formula plus the national SIFT, but are they to cut back to the average running costs of a general hospital plus SIFT, which is what the RAWP targets allow? The 45 Sample Hospital Formula gives an estimate of the costs of running a modern hospital. The RAWP estimates used in calculating targets, on the other hand, are a mixture of old and new hospitals.

This means that the revenue allocated by RAWP is insufficient to fund the running of a modern hospital. This problem is a particularly difficult one for teaching areas under current policies where students are being trained to work in a modern hospital.

It seems anomalous to train students in standards lower than those of a modern hospital, but if those standards cannot be afforded then it would seem that they ought to be redefined. What is remarkable is that the 45 Sample Hospital Formula estimates, together with the SIFT, do seem to come close to covering the costs of teaching, research and the whole range of treatments given at London teaching hospitals. The cuts based on the RAWP methods may create the necessary climate for a reappraisal of hospital services, but the methods provide no basis for resolving this problem. What seems to be required is a much more thorough examination of what standards of care ought to be provided at a modern hospital in terms of what we can reasonably afford to make available on a national basis. And we also ought to attempt a planned development of those standards that relate advances in medicine to future resources. This would give a better basis for decisions on how doctors should be trained, and the kind of standards and developments that they should expect to experience in their working life. Such examination and developments are necessarily matters for the longer term. They do, however, seem crucial if we are to move beyond the barren and frustrating clash of ideologies of excellence versus equity in which the controversy over the London teaching hospitals now appears to be trapped.

For the immediate future other issues are being explored which can reduce the discrepancy between the targets and actual expenditures of the teaching areas. The targets may be increased by better estimates of the high-cost specialties provided at the teaching hospitals. (An estimate of these costs for the Comptroller and Auditor General put these at only £3m for all the London teaching hospitals, so the relief from this refinement in the accounting for cross-boundary flow may turn out to be of little significance.[33]) And costs may be reduced by concentrating the development of expensive specialties (e.g. cardio-thoracic surgery).

Under past funding practices it seems likely that the London hospitals had the opportunity to develop expertise in expensive parts of medicine – perhaps too many. The danger of continuing current policies is that cuts could result in destroying well-established research teams which will be difficult if not impossible to replace. A problem here is to be able to distinguish between what ought to be preserved and developed and what ought to be rationalised. The concern about the present methods and organisational structure is that neither is designed for making this vital distinction.

Central Guidance and Local Discretion

There is a rather loose link between the Cabinet's allocation of public expenditure for its various purposes, and the decisions by Health Authorities on the details of expenditure.

Health Authorities are responsible for making decisions on policy, and therefore on expenditure, within the limits of instruction or guidance by Health Departments and their ministers, and within whatever expenditure limits are set. But the latter are single-block figures for revenue expense and for capital expense, with some elasticity between the two and between expenditure from one year to the next (see Chapter 11). Allocations for a special purpose are sometimes announced, with governmental authority: the Budget of April 1978 included £50m (in 1978–9) for specific improvements in services to patients. These were to vary from place to place but there would be, for example, extra resources for the full opening of newly completed hospitals, facilities to cut waiting lists, more staff to help care for the elderly and handicapped, and over 400 extra kidney machines. Earlier there had been substantial allocations for additional construction work and for the establishment of specially secure units for disturbed and violent patients; a report in the *Observer* for 27 May 1979 claimed that little of this money had been spent for the stated purpose.

The present system of complete delegation of decision from departments to authorities cuts across such special allocations, except where the department procures goods (e.g. kidney machines) and gives them to Health Authorities. As a result, the results intended by ministers – at the expense of the programmes or of the taxpayer – may not be achieved: authorities may simply take the money and use it at their own discretion. We conclude that allocations for specific purposes should not be made unless the payments are going to be controlled and audited. It may sometimes be right to allocate additional general funds, but this should be openly stated.

Resource Allocation in the UK

We have highlighted weaknesses in the RAWP approach in terms of guiding allocations to areas and districts. We consider finally the possible consequences of applying equalisation policies to the different countries of the UK.

The Public Expenditure White Paper published in January 1979 includes tables which give comparative expenditure in England, Scotland and Wales on health and social services.[34] This, together with the details of the Northern Ireland programme, enables us to compare expenditure per capita in the different countries. We have used the actual populations for 1977 and the forecast population for 1981 to give actual expenditure per capita in 1977–8 and planned expenditure forecast per capita in 1981–2:

Table 8.3: Expenditure Per Capita on Health and Personal Social Services in the Countries of the UK

Country	Population 1977 1,000s	Expenditure per capita in 1977–8 at 1978 survey prices	SMRs UK=100 1977 Male	Female	Planned expenditure forecast per capita in 1981–2 at 1978 survey prices £
England	46,351	142.4	98	98	156.9
Scotland	5,196	172.8	109	106	193.2
Wales	2,768	147.3	105	105	160.3
N. Ireland	1,537	175.7	115	114	198.1

Sources: Expenditure data from *The Government's Expenditure Plans, 1979– 80 to 1982–83,* Cmnd 7439 (HMSO London, 1979), Tables 4.5.1, 4.5.2 and 2.15; and population data from *Regional Statistics*, No. 15, (HMSO, London, 1979).

This analysis reveals striking variations and curious planned development of expenditure. There seems to be no simple explanation why Scotland should continue to receive significantly higher funding than either England or Wales. (Northern Ireland, given its separation from the mainland, and its small population, is a special case.) We can push this analysis further by comparing expenditure per capita of Wales, Scotland and N. Ireland with that of English regions. The expenditure per capita in this analysis (Table 8.4) is lower than in Table 8.3 because it only includes expenditure by Health Authorities (expenditure by

Table 8.4: Expenditure Per Capita in 1976—7 by Country and Regional Health Authorities

Country/Region	Population 1,000s mid—1977	Expenditure per capita Revenue	Capital	Total
		£m at 1976—7 outturn prices		
RHAs				
Northern	3116.0	91.5	8.0	99.6
Yorkshire	3571.9	91.8	6.4	98.2
Trent	4537.1	83.1	10.0	93.0
East Anglia	1827.4	86.8	7.0	93.8
N.W. Thames	3432.4	115.8	5.3	121.2
N.E. Thames	3695.8	110.6	6.6	117.1
S.E. Thames	3562.8	112.8	6.6	119.4
S.W. Thames	2855.1	109.5	9.0	118.4
Wessex	2661.0	88.5	6.8	95.3
Oxford	2237.1	87.6	6.9	94.5
South Western	3181.8	91.0	6.5	97.4
West Midlands	5154.3	86.9	5.5	92.3
Mersey	2475.7	98.5	9.7	108.2
North Western	4042.9	95.3	6.6	101.9
England	46,391	97.6	7.2	104.9
Wales	2,766	102.1	6.7	108.7
Scotland	5,206	107.6	7.8	115.4
N Ireland	1,537	125.8	9.5	135.3
UK	55,886	100.7	7.3	108.0

Sources: *Regional Statistics*, No. 15 (HMSO, London 1979), and DHSS.

local authorities on personal social services is excluded).

Just taking Health Authorities' expenditure per capita it would seem that Scotland ought to be subjected to similar constraints on growth of resources as the Thames regions. The Thames regions may expect revenue increases of about 0.5 per cent from 1979—80 to 1982—3, and no growth in their capital allocations.[35] Scotland on the other hand may expect percentage increases in total expenditure (capital and revenue) from 1979—80 to 1982—3 of about 1.5 per cent per annum.[36]

Of course crude population data alone are not an adequate basis for analysing expenditure in terms of equity: the various working parties have gone beyond these to include elements which attempt to take account of morbidity, cross-boundary flow and costs of teaching. (And Scotland is in a similar position to the Thames regions in its heavy teaching responsibilities: a fifth of all medical students trained in the UK are trained in Scotland.) It would seem unlikely that current methods of accounting for teaching and other refinements used by RAWP (on morbidity and cross-boundary flow) and by SHARE (on dispersion of population) would significantly affect Scotland's position. We consider that the relative figures should be better known. It is hard to see how the different treatment of the Thames regions and Scotland is justified on the basis of moving towards equitable allocation of resources for health care in the UK.

Notes

1. Lewis Carroll, *The Hunting of the Snark* (Chatto and Windus, London, 1953, 5th imp.).

2. Department of Health and Social Security (DHSS), *Sharing Resources for Health in England,* Report of the Resource Allocation Working Party (the RAWP Report) (HMSO, London, 1976).

3. Ibid., pp. 11,81 and 84.

4. Carroll, *The Hunting of the Snark.*

5. DHSS, *Health and Personal Social Services in England, DHSS Planning Guidelines for 1978/79,* Health Circular HC (78) 12 March 1978.

6. RAWP Report, p. 5.

7. Ibid., p. 8.

8. Ibid.

9. Ibid., p. 81.

10. Ibid., p. 82.

11. M.J. Buxton and R.E. Klein, *Allocating Health Resources: A Commentary on the Report of the Resource Allocation Working Party,* Royal Commission on the National Health Service, Research Study No. 3 (HMSO, London, 1978).

12. RAWP Report, p. 7.

13. Buxton and Klein, *Allocating Health Resources,* p. 6.

14. RAWP Report, pp. 78–9.

15. DHSS, *Priorities for Health and Personal Social Services in England,* A Consultative Document (HMSO, London, 1976).

16. Radical Statistics Health Group, *RAWP Deals,* 1977.

17. RAWP Report, p. 121.

18. J.R. Perrin, R.G. Bevan, H.A. Copeman, J. Owen, *Management of Financial Resources in the National Health Service,* Royal Commission on the National Health Service, Research Paper No. 2 (HMSO, London, 1978), pp. 85–102.

19. *Report of the Committee of Enquiry into the Cost of the National Health Service* (the Guillebaud Report) Cmd 9665 (HMSO, London, 1956), pp. 270–1.

20. *Report of the Royal Commission on Medical Education 1965–68* (the Todd Report) Cmnd 3569 (HMSO, London, 1968), p. 198.

21. Ibid, p. 172.

22. *Report from the Comptroller and Auditor General, Appropriation Accounts 1976–77,* vol. 3, Classes X–XV and XVII (HMSO, London, 1978), pp. xi–xv.

23. RAWP Report, p. 11.

24. Ibid.

25. Ibid., p. 13.

26. Ibid., p. 20.

27. Ibid., p. 84.

28. See T.C. Schelling, *The Strategy of Conflict* (Oxford University Press, London, 1960).

29. Ibid., pp. 21–52.

30. Ibid., pp. 53–80.

31. Todd Report, pp. 177–82.

32. RAWP Report, p. 52.

33. *Appropriation Accounts 1976–77,* vol. 3, Classes X–XV and XVII, pp. xi–xv.

34. *The Government's Expenditure Plans, 1979–80 to 1982–83,* Cmnd 7439 (HMSO, London 1979), Tables 4.5.1 and 4.5.2.

35. *DHSS Planning Guidelines for 1978/79,* Table 3.2.

36. *The Government's Expenditure Plans, 1979–80 to 1982–83,* Table 4.5.2.

9 PLANNING PRIORITIES

The NHS planning system was launched in 1976 with guidance from the DHSS on planning methods,[1] on priorities[2] and on resource assumptions. For those who tried to relate policies to available resources 1976 was a particularly trying year. It began in February with the Government's White Paper on public expenditure which announced cuts in planned growth.[3] But appraisal of the nation's resources showed that, short of an economic miracle, even these reduced growth rates could not be financed.[4] In July a package of cuts in public expenditure was announced, designed to reduce an expected overcommitment of resources. The resource assumptions issued to Health Authorities at the start of their first planning cycle were based on these plans. However, there were very serious pressures on the £ sterling, and in December, as part of a package agreed with the IMF, further cuts in public expenditure were announced.[5] Health Authorities were duly given revised lower-resource assumptions for their planning, although they were, by that time, half-way through the cycle to which those assumptions applied.

In our fieldwork for the Royal Commission it was this first planning cycle that we studied. Not surprisingly, a completely new process introduced into a recently reorganised NHS under these difficult circumstances was a long way from achieving its potential. It is not our concern here to dwell on the understandable shortcomings of the first cycle, especially since the second round of strategic plans that have been recently produced are a major improvement on those first attempts. There were, however, important misconceptions about the nature of planning which we do explore. Planning offers the NHS the potential for resolving the difficult problems of what to develop, what to maintain, what to restrain and what to stop. These choices are difficult, because even what is to be stopped will often have merit: but it is only by releasing these resources that other more effective or urgent developments can begin.

Relating Planning to Decision-making

The vital element of successful planning is its impact on improving decision-making. Unfortunately it is hard to know how planning has influenced decision-making, and there are no simple criteria for judging the quality of decisions about health care. Thus we never know the benefits of the considerable effort required to link planning to the taking of decisions. And judgements about the success of planning in achieving its most vital purposes are insubstantial and contentious. Those responsible for the production of plans are aware of these difficulties, and that their work may be judged by narrower criteria — whether the planner meets deadlines for the production of plans and the generation of data, or whether what is in the plan really happens. It is not easy to establish that planning did lead to better decisions.

The difficulties of planning with limited and uncertain resources, and requirements for consultation, make it difficult to produce plans in time, and resource uncertainty immediately undermines any hope that the future might be as planned. Not surprisingly therefore, in the first planning round, those responsible for producing plans complained of the difficulties of consultation within the planning timetable, and claimed that they could not plan unless resources were certain. The general approach was to produce an elaborate document that contained a good deal of data but was not costed, did not set priorities, and did not consider how to cope with an uncertain future.

The way planning ought to work is that the strategic plan lays out a statement of priority developments, and that these should be linked with budgetary allocations through the rolling operational plan. The plans are the basis for the formation of policy, and they are backed up by monitoring and budgetary control. If *priorities* are not set in strategic planning, the budget-setting continues incrementally, and planning has little impact. Since priorities are the crucial features of making decisions with limited resources, strategic plans that fail to set priorities do not lay out a strategy against which future developments can be monitored. And since the future is uncertain, plans have to consider *uncertainty* directly if they are to provide a useful basis for decision-making. If plans do not consider uncertainty at all, they will be discredited by inviting comparisons between what was planned and what actually happened. If strategic plans do not face up to the reality of having to decide on priorities for the use of limited resources, and cannot cope with uncertainty, they provide no real statement of policy, and important developments will be left to be decided in a piecemeal manner.

The main theme of this chapter is to explore the difficult process of setting priorities. In this process we use two different concepts of cost: the financial cost and the opportunity cost. The financial cost of a development is the total of money payments that a Health Authority will have to make for the resources used by that development.

The opportunity costs of a development are the opportunities forgone by that choice in terms of other options that cannot now be afforded. In setting priorities we can begin by comparing the financial cost of proposed developments with the financial resources that will be available. The total financial cost of these developments will normally exceed the additional finance that we might expect. The opportunity cost of those options finally chosen is the loss of the best option(s) (with the same financial cost) which has been rejected, as we saw on a national scale in Chapter 7. Fundamentally, planning is about assessments of opportunities forgone by current choices — including the choice to continue with existing activities. Financial costs are only a starting point: obviously the assessment of benefits is vital although more difficult. Unfortunately, even the relevant financial costs for planning purposes do not come readily from the financial information systems of the NHS.

Costing Plans

Costing by Care Group

The NHS financial information systems report costs of hospitals for the accounts, and of functional groups (e.g. nursing, catering, laundry, drugs) by which budgets are controlled. These data cut across the planning framework of care groups. The DHSS analyses revenue expenditure nationally by care group (in its programme budget) and indicates national priorities by care group both in terms of guidelines of service provision (i.e. staffing and/or beds) and distribution of expenditure. It is through the care-group framework that Health Authorities are expected to answer four fundamental questions of planning:

a. Where are we now? — i.e. taking stock.
b. Where do we want to be? — i.e. agreeing the strategy.
c. How do we get there? — i.e. means of achieving the strategy.
d. How are we doing? — i.e. monitoring progress.[6]

The DHSS has proposed some necessarily approximate methods that enable Health Authorities to answer these questions by deriving estimates of past and future revenue expenditure by care group. Two of these methods are based on annual hospital costs and information on patients treated at each hospital. Combining these two sources of data allows estimates of cost per case (preferably) or per bed to be derived for specialist hospitals for the mentally ill, the mentally handicapped, the geriatric and maternity services. In its simplest form this approach assumes these costs to be representative of the costs of treatment of patients in those care groups (whether in a District General Hospital or a specialist hospital). The costs of acute care (at District General Hospitals) are derived by substracting these groups from the total. This analysis provides the baseline data of costs for the most recent year for which actual costs are available. These methods can be extended to produce estimates of future costs by using the past estimate of cost per case (or per bed) in each care group and multiplying this estimate by the expected number of future cases (or beds). The DHSS asks for costs for an intermediate and the final year of the strategic planning period.[7]

These projections, together with the baseline analysis, provide a framework for answering in part the four basic questions in terms of expenditure by care group. The baseline gives actual expenditure. The strategy can be expressed in terms of intended future expenditure by care group both at the end of the period, and in terms of a path towards this goal. Expenditure can then be monitored against the path outlined in the strategy.

Developments in Financial Information Systems

When setting budgets it is relevant to know the goods and services that are likely to be required in the year, and the costs of providing them. The budget holder, to keep within his budget, has to know expenditure and commitments to date. For planning, one of the requirements is the analysis of expenditure by care group. It is attractive to think in terms of a system designed to produce information for budgeting and planning simultaneously. This is not necessarily the best solution — it might be too cumbrous — but we mention in Chapter 6 the promising developments in the new Standard Accounting System.

Financial costs are a measure of resource inputs. These inputs are revenue (which is mainly staff) and capital. There are no charges in the NHS for the use of capital (such as interest and/or depreciation or imputed rent). Refinements of current financial information systems will not routinely yield data either on capital that is currently being poorly used or the effects of new building on future running costs. Both kinds of data are vital to planning. With the limited growth available, Health Authorities must, if they are going to make best use of their funds, critically appraise their use of existing resources, which means special analyses and perhaps specially collected data. And because new hospitals are better equipped and therefore significantly more expensive to run than old hospitals treating the same number and type of patients, new capital can have a significant effect on future revenue.

It does not make sense to design an information system to attempt to produce these kinds of data on a routine basis: they are best estimated from *ad hoc* studies.

Whilst more accurate data on resource inputs can be useful, they are only one part of the data needed to make choices. We can see the need for more detailed costs by specialty, both in order to account properly for cross-boundary flow, in the methods of the RAWP, and so that Health Authorities in their operational planning have reasonable estimates of the likely costs of new consultant appointments. But because costs are only part of the relevant data there are limits to the effort worth expending on their production. We can illustrate this by considering the example of the costs of treating renal failure.

The Value of Costing

We have chosen the example of treatment of renal failure because it has been well researched[8] and because it appears to pose in an unusually acute form the problem of putting a value on saving life. There is a range of treatments which depend on the state of the patient and (in the case of transplantation) on the availability of suitable kidneys. The average costs of different treatments for renal failure have been estimated from the NHS accounting system. An exercise by the DHSS on an initial sample of 36 patients receiving transplants and 20 destined for home dialysis produced a range of annual costs from £1,000 to £10,000 per annum.[9] The cost depends on the nature of treatment and its success. Haemodialysis was estimated to cost £5,770 per annum at home and £10,800 per annum in hospital. Successful transplants are cheaper: support is still needed and was estimated to cost £1,250 per annum after the discharge from hospital. The success rate of transplants was approximately 60 per cent. The cost of a successful transplant was estimated to be £1,150, and of an unsuccessful transplant to be £4,930 (because of the intensive care needed following rejection).[9] Knowledge of the costs of treatment for renal failure is useful because we can estimate what would be needed to provide treatment for all who might require it. The prevalence of renal failure might be as high as 19 per 100,000, and of each 19 four might benefit from dialysis.[10] And the Office of Health Economics (OHE) has estimated the costs for treating those under sixty at £120–170m (depending on survival rates) and for all in need (including those over sixty) at as much as £350m.[11] Deciding how to ration treatment for renal failure at first appears to mean resolving the awesome prospect of putting a value on life. But we shall all die: the objects of treatment are to avoid premature death and to avoid unnecessary suffering. And we all voluntarily take risks of early death or suffering, in using the roads, in risky sports, in dangerous work or in smoking. The treatment for our example of severe illness, renal failure, is most properly appreciated as an attempt to reduce – or rather to defer – the risk of death. There is the complication that a person receiving dialysis may suffer considerable pain, discomfort and extremely unpleasant side-effects, such as having to take steroids. The clinician, in making decisions on treatment, will consider the quality of life that a patient may reasonably expect.

The need to make careful comparisons in this way applies more generally in decisions by the Government on other interventions that lower the risk of death. Gavin Mooney gives some illustrations of why there may be different values put on lives saved through the different interventions:

> the output of a cervical cancer screening programme is likely to be in terms of lives saved among middle-aged multiparous women of lower socio-economic classes whereas the Tufty Clubs, the National Cycling Proficiency Scheme and the Green Cross Code are only likely to affect children on the roads. The 'quality of life' on a kidney machine is likely to be very much lower than that of individuals saved from drowning. The future expectations of life of those who survived through the provision of coronary care units will differ markedly from that of lives saved through child-proof containers for medical prescriptions. Attitudes to death may vary according to circumstances – death from cancer may be thought more abhorrent (and consequently of greater value when avoided) than death in a road accident, which is frequently instantaneous; the prospect of accidental death 'at home' (Ronan Point, for example) may give rise to greater anxiety than that of death in an accident at work (construction workers, for example); and again the lone yachtsman stranded in mid-Atlantic is in a very different situation from that of the average family motorist going for a weekend jaunt in the British countryside.[12]

Other consequences of life-saving intervention have to be valued and balanced by those making decisions: perhaps the most notorious are the alleged interference with freedom through the wearing of safety-belts, or the random testing of the breath of motorists when the pubs close. There is a very wide implied range of values given to different interventions, even by the same person or authority. For example, safety measures taken to prevent death by changes in building regulations following the partial collapse of the Ronan Point high-rise block of flats have been estimated to cost a minimum of £20m per life saved, whereas another investigation of a method of preventing stillbirths suggested that this could be made standard practice for approximately £50 per life saved.[13]

Within the NHS, because of a lack of cost data on the treatments within acute care, there are no other costs with which to compare the estimates of the costs of treatment for renal failure. Even if these costs were known, the choices, as we have seen, would still be difficult to make. Much NHS treatment is directed not at reducing the risk of death but at making life more pleasant. This latter kind of treatment may or may not have to be reduced to make way for more of the former.

Within those treatments that are directed at reducing the risk of death and where costs can be measured — if, for example, treatment for cancer is found to be twice as expensive as renal dialysis — the conclusions are still not straightforward. It might be right to switch resources at the margin, but it would not be sensible to put all the resources into renal dialysis rather than cancer treatment on the grounds that more lives would be saved, nor even to make a straightforward proportional investment in these different kinds of treatment. Judgements ought to depend, at least, on the likely survival of the patient, the quality of survival, and on likely developments in the different treatments.

Whilst there are limits to the value of cost data in guiding decision-making, it is important that these data should be applied, and should give a sound basis for choice. But getting the relevant data for a critical appraisal of resource use is a wider process than extracting data from the existing financial information system, or from sophisticated developments of that system.

The Opportunity Cost of Capital

Health Authorities gaining revenue under DHSS policies of following the RAWP principles may lack the capital to make good use of the revenue they receive. Capital allocations are limited and uncertain. Health Authorities facing cuts in revenue because of current policies are seeking for means of reducing their expenditure. Each authority has therefore to examine its current use of resources: those who are gaining revenue to see whether they can deploy existing capital more intensively, and those who are losing revenue to see what closures and redeployment can secure the savings they have to make. There is no charge appearing in the accounts arising from the poor use of capital asset. But there can be high opportunity costs. For an authority gaining revenue, redeployment of capital may be the only way of making good use of that revenue for many years. For an authority losing revenue, redeployment of services and selling off hospitals that have been closed is a way of securing extra financial resources.

Revenue Consequences of Changes in the Use of Capital

The first point to make is that closing a hospital may result in only limited saving in revenue. The demand for treatment that was met by that hospital is likely to persist, and may have to be met elsewhere. Since nearly 75 per cent of revenue expenditure is on wages and salaries, significant reductions in revenue can only follow by reducing staff. But there is scope for redeployment, especially if closures are co-ordinated with the opening of new hospitals.

In changing the use of a ward the revenue consequences are the extra costs of the new services and the likely savings from stopping current services. Again the revenue savings may not, in practice, be significant unless the demand for current services can be accommodated elsewhere, without having to increase staff, and the current staff can be redeployed for the new services, or staffing levels reduced through wastage or even through dismissals.

Revenue Consequences of More Intensive Use of Resources

Health Authorities are encouraged to make more intensive use of their resources by reducing length of stay. This will probably allow more patients to be treated in a given year. Since cost per day of treatment is high initially and then declines, the higher throughput means replacing low-cost days with high-cost days, and running costs will increase. This is almost certainly a more efficient way of treating the *increase* in the number of cases than providing extra beds. But it does mean that if an authority is trying to *reduce* its expenditure, reducing length of stay (although providing a more efficient use of available resources) will mean an *increase* rather than a decrease in expenditure if more cases are treated.

If the purpose of reducing length of stay is not to increase throughput but to save costs, significant savings are only likely to accrue from redeployment of staff. The reduction in demand for nursing, drugs, food and laundry will of itself produce only small savings in terms of reduced purchases.

The Costs of Community Care

Reductions in length of stay may lead to more efficient use of hospital resources, but it is prudent to suppose that earlier discharge into the community leads to increased need for community care, and (where this need is not met) increased risk to health. This raises the more general point about the DHSS policy of encouraging care in the community both because it is cheaper and because it is more satisfactory for patients. In particular, the Consultative Document advocated developing community care for the elderly and the mentally ill. This policy is unconvincing because no analysis has been published which shows that community care is indeed cheaper. We do not know, for example, whether the costs borne by friends and relatives are included. As it stands there is a growing suspicion that, although the word 'community' has a comforting ring, it is used too readily (the patient may find less of a community in the outside world than within the hospital); and that, on the grounds of a move to community care, Health Authorities are making savings with detrimental effects on their patients.

Community care ought to be presented as a co-ordinated package giving benefits to patients who are able to live in their homes, and to Health Authorities, by allowing them to make better use of expensive hospital resources. But this package ought to be related to the analysis on which DHSS policies are based. Without knowing this analysis Health Authorities are seriously handicapped in implementing the policies based upon it, and both the analysis and the policies are open to the suspicion that they are not soundly based.

Setting Priorities By Care Group

The Contexts of Policy-making

Knowing relevant costs is only a first step in setting priorities. Getting these costs is difficult, as we have explained, but this exercise is still straightforward in comparison with the problem of choosing priorities. This requires bringing together costs and benefits and deciding what care is to be provided and what is to be forgone. This is necessarily a political and not an 'accounting' process, and depends on one's valuation of the various benefits. Planning of health services is inherently political, and decisions are formed by various types of pressure. Those who work in Health Authorities have their own ideas, as employees, on what should be provided. They may oppose changes which, although they may lead to greater efficiency or savings, mean that their work is altered adversely or they get sacked. There are general pressures for the involvement of workers in running many organisations, including the NHS. The local public are represented through Community Health Councils and through Health Authorities, and these bodies recognise the importance of local judgements about the development of a national service. In the end, however, the finance comes from the taxpayer through the Government. The Secretary of State is accountable to Parliament and the public for the NHS, and it is from his office that the setting of priorities begins.

The Status of the Priorities Promulgated by the DHSS

In promulgating national priorities, the Secretary of State is well aware that he can only offer broad guidance. Regions have to interpret these in the light of their circumstances, and set out their policies in their strategic plans. The Secretary of State can then decide on differences between national and regional policies: whether these differences are reasonable and can be approved; and whether such reasonable differences arise purely from local circumstances or mean that national policies ought to be modified.

The making of policy for the development of the NHS is a complex business involving several administrative layers and a variety of interest groups. The DHSS have to try to strike the proper balance of giving some direction to a national service. But they must avoid putting this in a form which is too detailed, because each Health Authority has to try to apply DHSS policies and take account of local differences in setting priorities for service development.

Guidance is offered by setting priorities in terms of the different care groups. There was an extensive general review in the Consultative Document of 1976[14] which laid out priorities across and within care groups. These priorities have remained basically unaltered since then, although they have been modified in minor ways in later publications.[15] Health Authorities are given an exposition of departmental priorities in three forms. There is the written text, an analysis by care group of expenditure on health and personal social services, and a table of guidelines of service provision. In the first planning round, Health Authorities tended to fasten onto the guidelines as the most straightforward way of translating departmental priorities to their own circumstances. This was a mechanistic approach which multiplied the guideline (of staff and/ or beds per thousand appropriate population) by the population of the authority requiring those services. This was an easy way out: following the written text required careful judgements, and the programme budget included local authority services. But the problem then arose that likely future resources would not fund developments that followed the guidelines. For example, the guidelines of the Consultative Document were used by one strategic plan as if they were a minimum requirement to be achieved during the period: where the authority was in excess of the guidelines no action was proposed, but it was suggested that all shortfalls should be made good. Although this plan was not costed, a calculation of a few minutes showed that the proposals required about twice the revenue increases that the authority was likely to receive. The plan recognised that its demand on resources was in excess of its likely allocation, and met this difficulty by demanding that its allocation be increased. This practice is unlikely to be tolerated in the current round. *The Way Forward* contained similar guidelines but emphasised their status:

> Therefore [they] represent broad *national* objectives. . . These are *not* specific targets to be achieved by declared dates, even at a national aggregate level. The 1979/80 projections are intended only to *illustrate* what might be achieved given provisional resources constraints.[16]

It is perhaps understandable that staff in Health Authorities have been puzzled by the use of two putative measures of need: the RAWP criteria used for resource *allocation,* and the guidelines used for resource *deployment.* They have complained that their allocations do not fund their guidelines. This confusion is due to a failure to appreciate the different purposes of the two processes. The RAWP targets guide allocation of limited resources between authorities. The planning guidelines are intended to guide the deployment of those resources within an authority. An area or region ought to be competent to make these latter judgements: but it is in a poor position to judge that it ought to be allocated more resources than it currently receives, because such judgements have to be resolved in terms of competing claims of other authorities.

There are, however, more fundamental questions about guidelines. Some of the misunderstanding may be similar to that we discussed in the earlier chapter on RAWP targets. In each case the DHSS has provided numbers around which negotiations can take place. There is no agreed basis from which theory can be developed to give precision in either the allocation or deployment of resources. It is often said that the DHSS guidelines have little or no theoretical basis. If the DHSS were to await the development of such a basis for the guidance it issues, it would probably have to give no guidance for a very long time – perhaps generations. The lack of a sound theoretical basis does not mean that the DHSS cannot intervene usefully in resource deployment. What matters is whether the status of the guidance is well understood and whether the focal points for negotiation are aptly chosen.

A general criticism of presentation is that, in the main, single figures are given whereas it may be more appropriate to indicate a permissible range. For example, the statement that the guideline for beds for mental illness and in-patients is 0.5 per 1,000 population[17] not only transmits that figure, but also suggests that there is a policy for uniformity (both nationally and locally), and it may therefore suppress innovation. Although there are caveats in the accompanying written text, these have less practical force than the figures in the table. If guidelines were expressed in terms of a range (for example, 0.4–0.6 psychiatric beds per 1,000 population) this might have a much greater impact than textual qualifications. A more fundamental point is that cases would be a better surrogate measure for planning purposes. The guidelines in terms of beds and staffing ought to provide a check on authorities' estimates of what they require to meet their expected caseloads, allowing for the existence of other facilities which will help to do the jobs – e.g. day places. Major discrepancies between requirements and the guidelines ought to be investigated. But if the object of planning is to use inputs efficiently, why promulgate guidelines in terms of beds? And since resources are inadequate to fund all the services that a Health Authority would provide if it were not constrained, guidelines also should indicate what ought to be forgone. Setting priorities means making both sets of decisions.

We now consider the nature of rationing of service development implied by the priorities of the DHSS.

The Priorities Promulgated by the DHSS

The priorities of the DHSS have remained unchanged since they were first promulgated in the Consultative Document of 1976:

> The central proposal in this document is that much of the available 'growth money' should be concentrated on services used mainly by the elderly and the physically handicapped, and mentally ill and handicapped, and children.[18]

It is commonly mistaken to interpret this statement as diverting resources towards long-stay care. But the Consultative Document emphasised the need of the elderly for acute care. The priority of putting more resources into geriatric services is a recognition of need that will arise from demographic change. The policies for the mentally ill[19] and the mentally handicapped[20] had been set out in White Papers issued prior to the Consultative Document, and all that was done in 1976 was to confirm those policies. One of the concerns about services for children was that the reduction in infant mortality in England was falling behind reductions made in other developed countries. Thus these priorities largely acknowledged known shortcomings in current services relative to future needs.

The care groups that were to be restrained were the general and acute hospital services and the maternity services. It was recognised that the growth envisaged for the former (1.2 per cent per year) would not meet all pressures for development, including the need to reduce waiting times. On maternity services a reduction in costs was proposed of two per cent a year: until 1976 the number of births had fallen sharply but the costs of maternity services had increased (between 1970 and 1973 the average cost per case rose by about six per cent a year in real terms).

In 1977 *The Way Forward* was published as the successor to the Consultative Document. It identified the main problem arising from the analysis of RHA strategic plans as 'a conflict, at least in the short term, between the priority for services for the mentally ill and mentally handicapped proposed in the consultative document, and the pressures on regions to invest in acute services.'[21] It stated that 'the question causing most concern (particularly among representatives of the medical profession) was the degree of restraint on further growth proposed for the general and acute hospital services'.[22] Departmental priorities have, however, remained unaltered since the Consultative Document. They were reaffirmed by *The Way Forward* and the planning circulars issued in 1978[23] and 1979.[24] These circulars stressed the link between the growth in the elderly population and the increasing demands for acute care. *The Way Forward* stated that RHA strategic plans had generally accepted the need to rationalise maternity services. The 1978 planning circular reported no implementation of this rationalisation: the birth rate had fallen but costs of maternity care had continued to rise. The 1979 planning circular announced a change in departmental policies because of the campaign to reduce perinatal mortality and handicap. This means increases in expenditure on hospital and community services and that 'expenditure on hospital obstetric services, instead of reducing as suggested in earlier guidance, should be expected roughly to maintain its level over the country as a whole, savings matching the costs of improvements'.[25]

The Debate over Priorities with Health Authorities

During our fieldwork we heard the view that the planning system was not useful because resources were determined by medical politics, and that planning could not affect this process. Thomas McKeown has criticised teaching hospitals for perpetuating a bias towards acute care:

> The effects of the tradition of the teaching hospitals on medical education have been profound. A medical service can be no more enlightened than the minds of the doctors who provide it, and the intellectual shutters are never again so widely open as during the period of training. Inevitably students acquire their concept of practice from the example provided by their teachers, and they leave the hospital aspiring to engage in the work they saw when training. It is for this reason that the isolation of teaching from some of the major health problems is so serious. A centre which excludes the mentally ill, the subnormal and many of the aged sick cannot be expected to provide doctors who care for them; and even the token admission of a few of these patients does not convey the idea that these are the largest and most formidable problems by which medicine is now confronted. It is therefore not possible to staff the major services unless the full range of problems and methods is displayed at the teaching centre where the work and interests of the future doctor are determined.[26]

If McKeown is right, and if medical politics do dominate decisions about Health Authorities' deployment of resources, then it seems that doctors are being trained to work in a different health service from that aimed for in the priorities of the DHSS. And the desired changes could only take place by radically altering the nature of medical education and not by the planning system. McKeown was drawing attention to one aspect of the problem. Perhaps teaching hospitals do provide the training their students want: for example, do many entrants aspire to work for the mentally handicapped? There are questions here about the preferences of society at large, of those who apply to and those who are selected for medical schools. McKeown suggests that potential students should be brought into contact with those parts of medicine which have long been neglected. One hopes that they will not be unduly put off by the conditions under which the elderly, the mentally ill and the mentally handicapped are often cared for. McKeown's proposal to remedy these problems is to construct new hospitals that can accommodate all kinds of patients and thereby overcome the problem of the isolation of those receiving long-stay care. This proposal means very large hospitals indeed (probably over 2,000 beds). Massive hospitals are difficult to run and may take years to build. The fundamental issue in providing long-stay care for those who will never again be independent is that the impact of medical treatment seems limited. The public money goes on making life as bearable as possible for these people. McKeown is advocating that we regard patients receiving this kind of care in the same way as an otherwise healthy individuals being treated in an acute episode. Even if this were sensible, putting patients with very different needs in the same building is an oversimple remedy for correcting an apparent bias against those who need long-stay care: the bias may remain and the gains from facilities may be outweighed by the losses caused by the size of the institution. We may all react against scandalous conditions, but it is not clear that the public wishes much more to be allocated out of the limited budget of the NHS to these groups.

Evaluating Benefits

Setting priorities entails the bringing together of costs and benefits. Whilst we can estimate costs by care group we lack data that indicate the benefits of treatment provided. High costs could indicate high quality and/or inefficiency. The NHS information on patient treatment records *throughput*, the passage of a patient through hospital, not *output*, the improvement in the condition of patients.

There are statistical and ethical problems in evaluating the efficiency and effectiveness of different kinds of treatment. This means that there is considerable uncertainty in knowing which improvements are attributable to medical intervention. Even if we knew this, we still have to measure the degree of each type of improvement, and make judgements about their relative values. A particularly difficult matter is how to assess the value of long-stay care. The state of the patient receiving treatment may not improve – indeed with the elderly and terminally ill there will be deterioration. What has actually been achieved is temporary alleviation. Rachel Rosser's research has been examining the problems of constructing a common scale for the severity of different states of disability and distress to provide a global measure for health output.[27] All such work is at an early stage of development and we are a long way from having a calculus of benefit to set alongside the costs of treatment. What is needed therefore is debate about rationing which is informed by expert judgement rather than premature attempts to quantify benefit. Clinicians are vitally important as experts in contributing to that debate, but the decisions on rationing are not exclusively clinical decisions, and ought to reflect wider values.

The Pressures on Acute and Long-stay care

Acute care can only gain resources at the expense of other services, and this would mean continuing neglect of those receiving long-stay care. This struggle is inherently frustrating for two reasons. First, putting more resources into acute care will not relieve for long the inexorable pressures on acute services. Second, as Alwyn Smith has expressed so clearly at a recent conference, the pressures on long-stay care will also increase because:

> The more that we prevent what we can prevent, and the more that we cure that which we can cure, the more we are left with that which we can neither prevent nor cure.[28]

The problem of allocating resources between the different care groups is almost inevitably biased towards acute care. For example, in its most emotional (if unrepresentative) form, the debate can be seen as denying life-saving treatment to ameliorate conditions for the mentally handicapped. Of course, not all acute care is of that highly dramatic kind, but the pressure of increasing waiting times gives continual dynamic to this debate, to bias it towards acute care.

The care group analysis provides the framework for constraining the debate and highlighting the shares being allocated to the groups which have suffered neglect in the past. The inadequacy of the framework is already apparent. There is going to be less growth available for acute care than will meet pressures for treatment. We can no longer look to the rationalisation of maternity services for extra resources. There does not seem to be scope for savings in the groups other than acute care (most of these are in any case priorities to which extra resources ought to be allocated). And therefore if acute care is to develop, choices must be made within that care group.

Problems of Rationalisation and Redeployment

Rationalisation is always difficult to effect in any organisation. The 1970 Conservative Government introduced Programme Analysis and Review (PAR) to appraise critically existing government expenditures. One senior civil servant is said to have remarked:

> Socrates was the first person to do a PAR. He went around Athens asking fundamental questions. Socrates was put to death. I do not want to do another PAR.[29]

That remark was published in 1974. And even now, some nine years after the introduction of PAR, there have been no dramatic changes in expenditure arising from the various reviews that have been undertaken. In a district, before rationalisation can become management policy it has to be agreed by each member of the District Management Team including the consultant representative (because management is by consensus). In some districts the consultant concerned wins the consent of his colleagues to these proposals. If he agrees to these proposals in the DMT without doing so he may be replaced because he is no longer seen as a representative by other consultants. If he is not prepared to negotiate nor commit the team to proposals that require negotiations, he is effectively putting a veto on the search for improved resource use. Without team backing the Finance Officer, for example, who has primary (but not exclusive) responsibility for pressing for more efficient resource use, is in a weak position to negotiate with consultants.

Problems of Planning Acute Care

The Lack of Cost Data

The general and acute care group accounts for 60 per cent of Health Authorities' revenue expenditure. But the available financial data are not in a suitable form to produce relevant costs of specialties. Functional budgeting means that specialty costs are not produced by the system of financial control. Since most types of acute care are provided in District General Hospitals there are no specialty hospitals whose accounts can be used to estimate costs of each specialty within acute care (though costs of care for the mentally ill and mentally handicapped, for instance, can be estimated in this way).

The Sources of Medical Advice

The current structure of the NHS is not designed to accommodate the clinical debate that needs to take place if we are to resolve the difficult questions of how to develop acute care with limited resources. The full-time medically qualified administrator, who might be expected to take the lead in organising the planning of acute care, is the community physician. The Grey Book expected a great deal from staff in these posts — expectations which have not been met, in part because of the shortage of suitably qualified staff. And it is unrealistic to expect those now in community medicine in the reorganised NHS to take a leading role in planning hospital services when they have spent most of their working lives in local authorities.

The medical advisory committees of the reorganised NHS were established to overcome the weaknesses of 1948, not the economic and social problems of 1979: they are focused on bringing together general practitioners and hospital doctors. Committees of this kind do not appear to be equipped to debate the complex problems now facing the development of hospital services.

The Organisation for Planning

The problems of planning acute care are strategic: the adjustments to be made require an extended time span. Yet the strategic planning of acute care is one of the major weaknesses of the reorganised NHS. In a multi-district area the team of officers includes no clinicians and is advised by the Area Medical Advisory Committee. That committee is ill-organised to give advice on acute care; and the Area Medical Officer, as a community physician, may not be expected to speak for clinicians. (The Grey Book does not pursue this point because it envisaged strategic planning originating at district level. It is at that level that it makes it clear that the community physician is not expected to speak for clinicians.) Clinical involvement is focused at district level, and it is hard for areas to bring together these local views to formulate a coherent strategy for the area. In single-district areas the complexities arising from the organisation structure are removed, but the administrative staff are heavily burdened with operational duties and may have little time to give to the preparation of plans (the two single-district areas we visited supported this hypothesis).

How Decisions Might be Taken

We can speculate about how decisions on acute care might be taken. It would seem difficult to formulate strategies within acute care at area and regional level via advisory committees, and by guidance from community physicians at those levels. Therefore we can expect decisions about acute care to be formulated, at least in the first case, by districts. The roles of areas and regions might be to indicate available resources for acute care in their plans, and to leave the detailed allocation of these resources to be formulated by districts subject to review by areas and regions.

The difficulties needing to be overcome before adopting a planning process of this kind are that, without themselves preparing strategic plans, districts would need to take a strategic viewpoint, and that regions and areas have so far no framework within the planning system to review developments in acute care. The DHSS would also need to acquire more background about developments of acute care than it gains from its present meetings with regions, and from regional plans.

The Weaknesses of the Reorganised NHS

The reorganised NHS and the new planning system are focused on making decisions on other than acute care. This omission extends down to planning teams at district level (Health Care Planning Teams/District Planning Teams) which have only exceptionally been established for the acute care group. This makes it especially difficult for the consultant representative on District Management Teams (DMTs) because he has to speak for and to hospital doctors without an adequate organisational structure for this dialogue.

We consider it urgent to resolve the current problems in planning acute care. Hospital doctors have no framework, no cost data, and an inadequate organisational structure for providing medical advice. Yet they have to resolve the critical problems of deciding how to use the scarce resources which will not provide enough to meet demand. If this problem is not tackled, consultants in the NHS will be alienated because they see conditions getting continually worse with no opportunity of taking action to resolve the problems that they face. Predictable responses will be demands for more resources, but it is not realistic to expect a significant increase in resources going to the NHS as a whole. Under these circumstances, the struggle over the distribution of those resources will become more intense and deeply frustrating.

Towards Resolving the Crisis of Acute Care

The Nature of the Problem

Although the reorganised NHS and the planning system are ill-equipped to resolve the problems of acute care, changes in organisational structure and the details of planning will not of themselves provide the key. What is at stake here is not a purely local problem affecting the NHS in England but a general problem facing countries of the developed world. It was inevitable that in the end the potential demand for health care would, given continual advances in medicine, outstrip the available resources. While this development has been taking place there has been an increasing awareness within the medical profession of the need to provide only treatments which are effective. And now we are faced with the unenviable position of having not been able to afford to provide effective treatment to those who need it.

What is now needed is a complete reappraisal of the practice of medicine under resource constraints. The casual devices of rationing by price or by location have been rejected as unfair: the UK abandoned rationing by price in 1948, and since the early 1970s there has been a movement towards geographical equity. This must mean rationing of services: deciding what is to be provided and what is to be forgone. And the need to make these decisions becomes more pressing with advances in new kinds of treatment for known diseases and in changes in the definition of illness. These developments again force a new perspective on rationing. In the past, for example, people died from renal failure because there was no known effective treatment: now we have effective treatment, but people still die because of shortage of resources. The explosive and, in some cases, highly expensive advances in medicine necessarily mean that we have to select those treatments which we are prepared to finance.

At the inception of the NHS, promises were made to the public that equal access to health care would be available, and to doctors that their clinical autonomy would be preserved. Resource constraints have always impeded clinical practice. The shortage of resources (relative to what could be used) is likely to increase, and there is a genuine and difficult problem in seeing how public policies about priorities can best be knitted into the individual clinician's autonomous relationship with his patient. This demands much constructive thought and debate. The problem is to decide how resource constraints should bite. This is now done implcitly by queueing and by doctors having to decide how to ration the resources at their disposal. Clinical autonomy can apply unlimited resources only if we as taxpayers are prepared to meet the costs of all available treatments. If, however, we are only prepared to finance some of the available treatments, it is unreasonable to place the burden of rationing solely on the doctors who treat us: likewise they may have to care for patients without having the ability to call on all the treatments they would like to apply, following decisions by responsible authorities. Planning has the potential as a process of open government of enabling authorities and the public to give broad policy guidance on where, having had advice from clinicians and others, they believe resources should be restrained.

Lord Beveridge argued in 1942 for freedom from want by better distribution of income from the times when we are working, to the times when we are unable to work.[30] In terms of health services the problem is that there is a limit on the resources we are prepared to contribute to treatment of people who are sick, which is less than the cost of the treatments which are clinically appropriate. But the magnitude of this problem is little understood. We have no model that gives a dynamic account of the generation of sickness in the community, and what this would entail in terms of a capacity of health and other services to prevent or treat that sickness. And we cannot reasonably expect such a model, given our current understanding, because there is no unequivocal definition of sickness. Even a definition in terms of remedial action will be a changing one because of changes in our understanding of illness and developments in treatment. We cannot therefore expect an exact or unchanging model of this kind, and certainly at present we must look for other solutions.

When comprehensive approaches are not possible, one has to seek for the most critical aspects of the problem, to see if they pose a clue. The greatest impending burden on the NHS is the treatment of the elderly. In terms of the redistribution argued for by Lord Beveridge, those in work are not prepared to finance all the treatment available for those who are retired. This problem of a shortage of resources is one that we may all reasonably expect to face when we are old – although its intensity is affected by the population balance between the numbers in work and the numbers who are retired. The problem can be seen as agreeing on a humane approach to rationing care for the elderly. Rationing can take different forms: queueing for diagnosis and treatment, denying treatment because it is too expensive, or lowering its quality. One possible approach is to consider at what point diminishing marginal returns set in for the elderly: we cannot reverse the ageing process. A second approach is to regard waiting lists as a fair way of rationing resources which are too scarce to be available to all without delay. The point at issue is not new. Such rationing is already done implicitly. Our argument is that these choices should be decided openly, and recognised as a necessary consequence of the resource constraints facing the NHS.

We now consider new directions needed to enable these choices to be made through planning.

Promulgation of Policies by the DHSS

As they stand, DHSS priorities recognise the pressing demands on future services by the elderly but provide no basis for resolving how these can be met with limited resources. The care-group framework is of limited use in analysing the problem, since much of the treatment given to elderly patients falls within the acute care group. We recognise that, in one sense, age is a poor discriminator because good health does not of course stop at a certain age; nor are degenerative diseases solely the plague of the elderly. Nevertheless, age is used as one of the criteria in rationing treatment for renal failure. And as resource constraints bite more severely, age is likely to become increasingly important in the rationing of acute care.

If the DHSS is to take lead in giving direction on rationing acute care, it seems that a different framework has to be developed for the debate over priorities that is needed. It is vital to subdivide the acute care group. Given the problems of rationing care for the elderly it might be most helpful to structure that subdivision to help us to make those decisions. A structure that enabled us to see what we were spending on the elderly and that could relate these costs to descriptions of the care given seems essential. It is not clear what the most suitable structure would be. Disaggregation by specialties, for example, although appealing in terms of deriving cost data, may not be the most appropriate. It may well be most useful to refine the general concept of the care-group approach down to types of elderly patient and the combinations of treatments they receive.

Planning by Health Authorities

Health Authorities need to devise ways for the clear formulation by clinicians of the nature of choices to be made in the rationing of acute care. There appears to be no adequate forum for this debate within the current advisory structure. The reorganised NHS focused on clinical involvement at district level. But the hard choices to be made in acute care are not a local matter. They are fundamental to policies of RHAs (and indeed of the NHS as a whole). What needs to be done is to bring together, with regions, representatives of the specialties within acute care together with qualified community physicians, who will be respected by hospital consultants, to work out rationing policies. These policies need to be debated: within the region and its areas and districts; with the DHSS; and with the public through Community Health Councils.

Medical Education

It is worth indicating here some of the problems emerging from the potential conflict between the excellence aspired to in medical education and the rationing that is an intrinsic part of service provision. For example, a paper published in 1978 by the University of London entitled *The Clinical Resources Required by General Medical Schools in London*[31] included a section on 'The Relevance of High Standards'. The first paragraph began by emphasising the importance that 'students should see the highest standards of care, both in hospitals and outside them' and ended by mentioning that 'training should not be related only to the individual patient, but also to a defined and recognisable community such as a District or Area'. It is not possible to find resources to apply 'the highest standards' (in the sense of the resources of a teaching hospital) to the community at large. Medical students are trained to ration available resources in the course of treating patients. But this is only one part of the rationing process. It is also vital that clinicians take part in allocating the resources which act as constraints on their work in treating patients. Medical students now have lectures in sociology and epidemiology, which give some conceptual basis for the more difficult problem of rationing resources to the community at large. But there are limits to how much of this material can be included in an overburdened medical curriculum. There may be scope for further training in broader approaches to rationing when doctors have achieved senior positions in hospitals or in general practice. The current shortage of community physicians is a natural consequence of a medical education which is designed to train clinicians with emphasis on the individual patient. This traditional emphasis may continue to be the most appropriate at that stage of a doctor's training. Clinicians may become interested in a community-based approach later in their careers, and some may wish to take up part or full-time posts which enable them to plan service development for the community. There are other possibilities: a consultant psychiatrist, for example, may be interested in developing expertise in developing psychiatric care for the community, while still practising as a psychiatrist. The creation of such posts is one possible long-term solution to the shortage of community physicians. Another quite different solution might be to regard community medicine as a possible career for people who have not been trained as doctors but who have been taught medical knowledge relevant to planning services for a community.

Planning for Uncertainty

If plans are to provide a useful basis for decisions they not only have to set priorities within limited resources, but to consider how to cope with changes in those resources, in the population, in values and in medical technology. We can understand the anguish that resulted from the change in resource assumptions half-way through the first planning round. No one expects planners to have to cope with changes like that as an integral part of planning, but planners must expect changes to be made in resources made available to the NHS over the ten-year period of strategic planning. We begin by describing the different processes which each contribute to the resource uncertainty with which Health Authorities and Health Districts have to cope.

The Origins of Resource Uncertainty

Allocations by the Cabinet

It has been argued that the NHS ought to have a guaranteed allocation, and thereby be insulated from the consequences of the turbulent environment through which the Government attempts to steer the economy, and from the vicissitudes of successive performances by their own (and other) spending ministers in the Cabinet. This, if granted, would of course give the NHS the certainty of resources which many would find of value. It is therefore worth speculating on what the NHS might achieve by a concordat of this kind, what it might mean, and the feasibility of its being achieved.

A guaranteed certain growth might mean a lower total rate of financial growth than would be likely to be secured by successive Cabinet decisions — whether the annual PESC allocations or counter-cyclical extras (see below). This would mean that the Secretary of State would have to forgo extra resources if the Government decided to increase their allocations of public expenditure to a greater volume than that assumed at the time the concordat was agreed. It would also mean that in a ministerial shuffle a new Secretary of State would not be able to reopen the decision and attempt to secure an increased share for the NHS in Cabinet debate: otherwise the concordat would mean little or nothing. However low the guaranteed growth, the concordat would come under stress during economic crises. The tension of Cabinet debates over reaching agreement on where cuts should fall might be intolerable if NHS expenditure were allowed to continue its smooth increase whilst other programmes took the total burden of the necessary cuts. It is therefore unlikely that the Chancellor, or the other spending ministers, would agree to any concordat that would be useful to the NHS management.

One might maintain that the suggestion of a concordat derives from an (understandably) parochial view of the NHS. The economic crises which result in cuts in public expenditure are sadly all too predictable. What is required if fluctuations in programmes are to be minimised is that the Cabinet should limit the growth so that it does not exceed a reasonable expectation of the rate of growth of the economy as a whole. This was the rationale of the Plowden Committee in 1961, and (at various times since) it has been reiterated with conviction by successive governments after having been chastened by severe economic crises and the traumatic consequences of cutting back on public expenditure plans. In the years leading up to the crisis the principle is nominally upheld, but only by straining credibility with over optimistic assessments of future economic growth. The difficulty in maintaining responsible action by spending ministers collectively is that as each minister 'fights his corner' they may affect not only the share of their programmes but the total of public expenditure. The last Labour Government overcame this problem by a two-stage process: the Cabinet first agreed on the total and then proceeded to agree on how this was to be distributed. And additional control over changes from these agreed plans was (and probably still is) exercised by setting aside a sum for the Contingency Reserve in these plans. All increases had to be taken from this total. This meant that later, incremental decisions could not undermine the strategy on which the original plans were based. Nevertheless, any such discipline is self-imposed by the Cabinet and will only last as long as the Cabinet as a whole agrees to its imposition. The general attitude of a Prime Minister is of enormous importance here.

Revenue Allocations by the DHSS

When allocations depended on the level of earlier allocations, the swings in any region's resources depended only on variations in growth money available nationally (after allocating Revenue Consequences of Capital Schemes (RCCS)) including the effects of crisis cuts. Regions did not have to worry about financing the running of their new hospitals, since they received RCCS for this. Now they have to consider how to run new hospitals from their revenue allocations, which are themselves uncertain. Under current policies the Thames regions may only expect 0.25 to 0.5 per cent annual growth over the next ten years.[32] This means that swings in growth available to the NHS in England are shared between fewer regions than formerly, and these regional variations will be greater than the national swings arising from central decisions on public expenditure. There is a ceiling on the growth a region may receive: the DHSS planning guidelines[33] stated that no region could expect revenue in excess of three per cent per annum. In these guidelines the DHSS has given average annual rate of growth for each region subject to the caveat that these may vary by a third either way. This means, for example, that the South Western region's increase for instance over the next ten years (2.1 per cent) could vary between 1.4 and 2.8 per cent. Because these rates are at compound interest they translate into possible total increase lying between 15 and 32 per cent over the ten-year period, which in revenue in the final year would range from £37m to £78m (at 1978–9 forecast out-turn prices). Another way of looking at the revenue uncertainty of that region is that they are virtually certain of a growth rate of 1.4 per cent per annum (£37m) and they can expect extra growth up to an extra 1.4 per cent per annum (another £41m).

This wide range of uncertainty over revenue growth is not only due to sharing this growth according to current estimates of need. A further complication arises from the use of RAWP 'targets' when these targets also move. Incremental allocations gave stability to the regional allocations, and have been properly criticised for their slow response to population changes. Current policy of taking account of distance from RAWP targets in making these allocations does relate these to population changes in an attempt to respond to changes in need for health care. But, in so doing, uncertainty about future population means uncertainty about the basis on which regional allocations are made. The problem is not merely one of changes in the population of a region (which is affected by births, deaths and, importantly, migration). Changes in the structure of the population and in Standardised Mortality Ratios also affect the targets. The latter can be particularly significant subregionally because the RAWP method of allocation assumes that the need for revenue is linearly proportional to SMRs. Even at regional level we heard of a target changing by £2m because of changes in its population data.

Revenue Allocations by Regions and Areas

As the allocations of growth money by the DHSS between regions — which takes account of the distance from RAWP targets — means that regions have greater uncertainty over their growth in revenue than England as a whole, so does the similar policy followed by Health Authorities exacerbate uncertainty in resource allocations to areas and districts. Regions are in a similar position to the DHSS in having to make judgements about ceilings and floors of movement of areas toward their targets. It seems likely that the resource change that areas may have to cope with will be greater than those of regions. Within each region it is likely that some areas will face cuts or be allowed little or no growth, while the other areas will take the lion's share of available growth. This means that changes in growth money nationally will affect most dramatically areas and districts further below their RAWP targets.

Although the Thames regions are not liable to major changes in growth in revenue, areas and districts still face considerable uncertainty in their future allocations. Given the limited growth that Thames regions can expect, the extra resources that below-target areas may receive will depend on cuts made on the inner London areas. These cuts will have to be continuously negotiated, and their outcome is extremely uncertain. Such decisions are not merely matters of regional or area policy but are of national concern. What is relevant here is that for hospitals or others working within the Thames regions there will continue to be considerable uncertainty over resources, although the origin of this uncertainty is different from those which apply in other regions in England.

Problems in Making Capital Allocations

The allocations of capital to the NHS as a whole are much more liable to changes on macro-economic and financial grounds than are the revenue allocations. The DHSS has not as yet used the RAWP criteria for capital as the basis on which future capital allocations will be made, but it may do so. Capital allocations would then be related to targets based on forecast population (for five years ahead) weighted for age, sex and SMRs. It is clearly essential that capital provision ought to reflect future needs and therefore relate to future populations. But combining the national uncertainty over the total available to the NHS in England, together with distributing this according to need as indicated by moving targets, does mean considerable uncertainty for Health Authorities in the capital they might receive. And because capital feeds through into demands on revenue this uncertainty over capital would affect the whole of an authority's planning.

Key Points for Health Authorities

Changing Resource Decisions

The first point to be made is that whatever the Cabinet decides about *planned* levels of expenditure the growth in *actual* allocations to the NHS is likely to be in the long run about the same as that of the economy as a whole. A Government may plan faster rates than the economy can withstand but will then be forced to make crisis cuts to bring public expenditure back into line. The consequences for the NHS of the Government's overoptimistic assessments of economic growth are changes in the *phasing* of growth money, not in *long-term totals.* Perhaps Health Authorities could approach planning as stating priorities in terms of phasing claims on resources. This approach suggests that cuts and increases from the expected resource growth can be seen as accelerating or retarding the progress of those developments with lower priorities. If this is a workable basis for planning, it should minimise the need to renegotiate priorities for changes in resources. But it may prove extraordinarily difficult to distinguish priorities between the few developments that can be afforded within limited resources.

The Value of Counter-cyclical Measures

Counter-cyclical measures are short-term actions designed to increase employment in this country. They do not include increasing employment in the public sector: this is a long-term and a not a short-term measure — one cannot recruit teachers in a slump and sack them in a boom. A general stimulus to demand, such as reduction in taxation, may do little to increase employment in this country, because the extra money may be spent on foreign goods. The Government has therefore tended to direct these short-term stimuli towards industries which — though with their share of structural problems — are suffering a particularly sharp drop in demand. The construction industry is one example.

One of the results of counter-cyclical measures has been the allocation of extra sums to Health Authorities for construction work: this gives extra resources but adds to uncertainty about the future as well. Some NHS staff told us that they were unable to make good use of such money granted at short notice: better use could have been made if this money could be used in a few years time. Such objections miss the point of counter-cyclical measures: if Health Authorities can use unemployed construction workers, then (putting it in terms of national finance) the cost of their labour is at most the difference between what they would receive as unemployment benefit and what they receive when employed; if those workers were to be used in, say, three years time, they would be taken from other employment. The underlying concept is that of opportunity cost: the cost of opportunities forgone by using resources for a particular purpose. The opportunity cost of a construction worker depends on what he would be doing if he were not employed by the Health Authority. It may well be that capital schemes produced at short notice are of less merit than those that could be produced given some years preparation. But not only would the benefit have increased in this time: so also would the opportunity cost.

Relating Health Resources to RAWP Targets

We argued in our report[34] against making short-term changes in allocations because of changes in RAWP targets. We discuss below the difficulties faced by Health Authorities because of conjunctural measures taken by the Government on economic grounds. In that case the difficulties can be justified, but short-term changes made solely because of changes in RAWP targets cannot be justified in the same way. We admit that there is virtue in using up-to-date information, but having to cope with sudden increases or cuts at short notice is unlikely to lead to the best use of available resources. In this case the opportunity cost of granting extra resources is the sudden cuts made by one authority, and the benefits are those that the gaining authority can secure by quickly arranging to spend its unexpected increases. Such changes would promote equality in money according to the RAWP criteria, but they would be unlikely in the short term to provide commensurate progress in equality of provision of health care: it is possible that the gaining authority may dispose of (at least some) of its unexpected increases in a spending spree at the expense of, for example, cutbacks in desirable maintenance work by the losing authority. The RAWP criteria are only surrogate measures, and were not seen by the working party as precise measures of need. There must therefore be limits within which short-term changes in RAWP targets should be followed by related allocations.

The argument we have advanced for stability in allocations only applies in the short-to-medium term. In the long term – certainly within the ten years of strategic plans – we would expect allocations by the DHSS to change following changes in population data. We therefore see the policy of allocating resources according to need (as measured by population data) as necessarily leading to greater uncertainty over resources.

Coping with Uncertainty

Much of the resource uncertainty originates in changes in capital allocations, but these changes affect revenue expenditure because new buildings bring increased running costs. An advantage of developing care in the community is that it is less vulnerable to changes in capital allocations.

Authorities still have to cope with these changes in capital. Where the purpose of a sudden increase in capital is to provide work for the unemployed in the construction industry, this might be achieved by commissioning extra maintenance work. Plans might therefore include a schedule of such work so that authorities can make use of capital money granted at short notice. It is of some value for authorities to have a number of small projects on the shelf to use grants of this kind, especially if design staff have time in between major projects, though at some risk that by the time the money is granted these projects may be out of date and no longer worthwhile.

The problem remains of coping with cycles of cuts and increases in capital during the building of a hospital. Over a ten-year period the total capital allocation may be as indicated in current DHSS guidance, but the flow of the capital money is likely to be uneven. What must be done is to design hospitals so that their construction can depend on the availability of capital funds, and so that when they are completed changes can be made in the use of wards. This might result in higher construction costs. A difficult balance has to be struck between the costs and benefits of flexible design.

Planning and Growth Money

Why is it that NHS staff still demand certainty over resources as a prerequisite for planning when reason and experience show this demand to be quite unrealistic? And given that uncertainty in planning is not limited to finance — priorities, medical technology, staff availability and population structure and movements are other uncertainties — why is it that this demand for certainty focuses on finance? There clearly are methodological problems associated with coping with uncertainty in terms of phasing the deployment of staff, capital and revenue. But before these can be faced there has to be a willingness to concede that planning involves exploration of the consequences of different resource assumptions. At the time of our fieldwork such willingness was exceptional despite exhortations from the DHSS to take account of uncertainty. A clue to this attitude — puzzling to the outsider — may be in the observation that for many in the NHS *planning is about growth money*. DHSS guidance is clear that planning ought to be about total resources and include a critical appraisal of the current use of resources. As long as planning focuses on growth money, resource uncertainty will threaten to undermine the exercise; and only when planning considers total resource use will this vulnerability be reduced. One of the problems here is linking planning and the setting of budgets. Normal, but not invariable, practice is to set next year's budget at last year's level of volume without challenge. Whilst planning provides the process of learning what has to be forgone in terms of new developments by not making savings on existing expenditures, the savings can only be realised through the budgetary process. In Chapter 11 we approach the task of introducing an appraisal of costs and benefits into budgeting in the NHS.[35]

Notes

1. Department of Health and Social Security (DHSS), *The NHS Planning System* (HMSO, London, 1976).
2. DHSS, *Priorities for Health and Personal Social Services in England*, A Consultative Document (HMSO, London, 1976).
3. *Public Expenditure to 1979–80*, Cmnd 6393 (HMSO, London, 1976).
4. See *Fourth Report from the Expenditure Committee, Session 1975–76* (HMSO, London, 1976).
5. See S. Brittan, *The Economic Consequences of Democracy* (Temple Smith, London, 1977).
6. DHSS, *NHS Planning System*, p. 8.
7. DHSS, *Draft Addendum to the NHS Planning System: Future Form and Content of Strategic Plans*, issued with a covering letter from Mr R. S. King to Regional Administrators, 11 January 1978.
8. See Herbert E. Klarman, John O'S. Francis and Gerald D. Rosenthal, 'Cost Effectiveness Analysis Applied to the Treatment of Chronic Renal Disease', *Medical Care*, vol. *VI*, no. 1 (1968), pp. 48–54; M. J. Buxton and R. R. West, 'Cost-benefit Analysis of Long-term Haemodialysis for Chronic Renal Failure', *British Medical Journal* 2, (1975), pp. 376–9; Joseph S. Pliskin and Clyde H. Beck Jr, 'A Health Index for Patient Selection: A Value Function Approach with Application to Renal Failure Patients', *Management Science*, vol. 22, no. 9 (1976), pp. 1009–21.
9. William Laing, *Renal Failure, A Priority in Health?* (Office of Health Economics, London, 1978).
10. M. McCormick and V. Navarro, 'Prevalence of Chronic Renal Failure and Access to Dialysis *Int. J. Epid.* 2 (1973), 247–55.
11. Laing, *Renal Failure*.
12. Gavin H. Mooney, *The Valuation of Human Life* (Macmillan, London, 1977), p. 75.
13. Ibid, p. 74.
14. DHSS, *Priorities for Health*.
15. See DHSS, *The Way Forward* (HMSO, London, 1977); DHSS, *Health and Personal Social Services in England, DHSS Planning Guidelines for 1978/79*, Health Circular HC (78) 12 (March 1978); DHSS, *Health and Personal Social Services in England, DHSS Planning Guidelines for 1979/80*, Health Circular HC (79) 9 (April 1979).
16. DHSS, *The Way Forward*, p. 21 (emphasis in original).
17. Ibid., p. 22.
18. DHSS, *Priorities for Health*, p. 27.
19. DHSS, *Better Services for the Mentally Ill*, Cmnd 6233 (HMSO, London, 1975).
20. DHSS, *Better Services for the Mentally Handicapped*, Cmnd 4683 (HMSO, London 1971).
21. DHSS, *The Way Forward*, p. 33.
22. Ibid., p. 28.
23. *DHSS Planning Guidelines for 1978/79*.

24. *DHSS Planning Guidelines for 1979/80.*

25. Ibid.

26. Thomas McKeown, *The Role of Medicine. Dream, Mirage or Nemesis* (Nuffield Provincial Hospitals Trust, 1976), p. 134.

27. Rachel Rosser and Vincent Watts, The Measurement of Illness, *Journal of the Operational Research Society*, vol. 29, no. 6 (1978), pp. 529–40.

28. See T. Rippington, CIPFA Seminar, *Health Economics*, vol. 4, no. 12, pp. 454–64.

29. H. Heclo and A. Wildavsky, *The Private Government of Public Money* (University of California Press, 1974).

30. Sir William Beveridge, *Social Insurance and Allied Services* (the Beveridge Report), Cmd 6404 (HMSO, London, 1942).

31. University of London, *The Clinical Resources Required by the General Medical Schools in London* (1978).

32. *DHSS Planning Guidelines for 1978/79.*

33. Ibid.

34. J. R. Perrin, R. G. Bevan, H. A. Copeman and J. Owen, *Management of Financial Resources in the National Health Service* (HMSO, London, 1978), p. 25.

35. For a review of information requirements for planning, its organisation in the DHSS Programme Budget, and discussions of the valuation of inputs and outputs, see J. W. Hurst, *Rationalizing Social Expenditure – Health and Social Services* in M. V. Posner (ed.), *Public Expenditure* (Cambridge University Press, Cambridge, 1977).

10 ALTERNATIVE FINANCING

Previously we have considered how the level of NHS funding is decided at government level, and how that funding is allocated (by RAWP and other criteria) downwards through the NHS tiers until spending authority eventually comes to rest in the 'functional budgets' of non-clinical managers (Chapter 4). Additional financial problems, and the constraints upon significant enlargement of NHS funding, have been explored in Chapter 7.

In this chapter we consider the question of alternative sources and methods of funding health care in Britain. It will be helpful if we take account of the experience of other countries in their use of alternative approaches to funding. In most other countries private medicine plays a much more important role than in Britain: when considering the total supply and funding of health care resources, it is essential to include consideration of the present and likely future role of private health insurance, and its possible implications for the NHS.

UK Health-spending Compared

The growth and scale of health care spending has been discussed in earlier chapters. The World Health Organisation, the OECD and various other bodies publish statistics on health service resources and costs that attempt to compare events in different countries. These statistics vary somewhat in their definitions and classification — and they cannot provide precise comparability despite attempts to correct for differences in health service structures, financing and statistical classifications. In particular, the line of demarcation between health services and personal social services varies from country to country; and also it is not certain that all countries' statistics manage to capture the total expenditure on private medical care (e.g. the private purchase of primary care and drugs). Moreover, published international statistics are always a few years out of date, and this is significant to the extent that health care expenditure has been growing quite rapidly in nearly all countries, but at different rates. Growth of spending on health in the UK would appear to be perhaps at the slowest rate experienced amongst the developed nations, with the possible exception of Japan (see Figure 7.4 and OECD statistics[1]).

Allowing for errors and variations amongst the comparisons published, it does appear highly probable that UK spending on health care is between one and two per cent below the proportion of available national income (whether measured as GDP or GNP) expended on health care by most other comparable countries. In round numbers this approximates to a lower annual expenditure of between £1,500m and £3,000m in the UK. Perhaps £2,000m represents a 'typical' difference in annual expenditure on health care as between the UK and other developed West European countries of similar population.

It is instructive to ask ourselves how it can be that the UK 'gets by' in health care whilst spending roughly 20 or 25 per cent less on health care than other countries: what comprises the £2,000m difference? Possible causes of the difference are as follows:

Possible Causes	Our Comments
a. Higher productivity in the NHS than in other countries.	There is some evidence that UK doctors and surgeons have above-average workloads, and that length of hospital stay is lower than in most countries, although not lower than the (high-cost) USA.[2]
b. Lower pay in the NHS than in other countries.	Medical, managerial, and scientific and technical staff are almost certainly relatively poorly paid in the NHS, but it is not clear that nursing and certainly other ancillary staff are (relative to other occupations in those countries) worse paid in the UK than in other countries.
c. NHS purchasing of drugs, supplies and equipment is more economical.	The monopsonistic power of the NHS (and DHSS) has held down prices of drugs and supplies, and of domestically produced equipment whilst growth of centralised stores management has contributed some savings.
d. The NHS has lower overheads.	NHS costs of administration are probably lower than in most countries — largely because costs do not have to be recorded, monitored, invoiced and collected for each individual patient, as in most other countries. Also the NHS does not pay interest on its capital, thus understating true costs by £500m or more per year.

e. The NHS has cheap or low standards.

We do not know of clear evidence on this, relevant to strictly medical standards. As regards the hotel aspects of hospital accommodation, and perhaps other aspects of patient facilities, it is almost certainly true that a more utilitarian and sometimes impersonal provision is supplied in the UK.

f. The NHS delivers a lower volume of health care (implying that the need or at least the demand for care is not met as fully as in other countries, or else that health care needed and/or de-demanded is less in the UK).

The NHS probably delivers an above-average volume of primary care, and probably an at-least-average volume of community care. It delivers a probably below-average volume of hospital medicine, and it certainly provides a lower volume of surgery than in many other countries. However, the need for, and benefit from, much elective surgery is anyway challenged (notably in the USA and Germany). Nevertheless, there do appear to be certain conditions for which the NHS does not supply a desirable volume of health care (e.g. renal disease and orthopaedic surgery for arthritis, etc.).

g. Public health care gives better value than private medicine (n.b. the UK share of private medicine in total health care is smaller than in most other countries).

The evidence is uncertain. Private medicine (as by analogy in the UK with NHS dentistry under the 'fee for service' payments system) may achieve high efficiency on routine procedures at least, yet may also exact high remuneration and profits more than offsetting the 'savings' from the high efficiency. Private medicine largely avoids queueing, but only by providing excess capacity with extra cost (e.g. notably in the USA[3]).

h. The UK system of financing the NHS direct from central government funds is more successful in controlling expendi-

There is no conclusive proof on this point, but it does seem likely that central funding can reduce expenditure on health care below the level of spending generated in systems more dependent

ture growth.

upon 'fee for service' financing – where both patients and doctors have greater influence over the amount of service delivered (sometimes with financial incentives for over provision – e.g. unnecessary surgery[4]).

Eight possible causes of lower relative spending on health care in the UK have been cited above. There may be other likely causes as well: for example, it can be argued that because affluence has grown more slowly in the UK in recent times, relative to other countries, we may be more reluctant than others – whether acting as individuals or by collective will exercised through government – to increase our health care spending substantially under present conditions. Without extensive research it would be impossible, we feel, to attribute any precise shares of the UK's overall £2,000m 'saving' on health care expenditure, against the suggested causes listed. What does seem probable, however, is that the common factor lying behind all the likely causes – good or bad – is that the NHS is a large, national system, funded centrally by allocation and budgets firmly specifying maximum expenditure (by cash limits) irrespective of demand (except in the case of family practitioner services, which are not cash-limited). If this is correct, then the burden of proof that better-value health care can be obtained must be placed upon the shoulders of those who would alter the present method of funding the NHS, or alter the balance between UK public and private health care provision. If the alterations would increase the total costs (by at least £3,000m, if we were to match the leading countries), then the protagonists of change must clearly specify what additional benefits the British people are to gain, for what additional cost. Here bear in mind that if the present provision of health care were widely accepted as severely inadequate, there is at the present time nothing to prevent public opinion, politicians and government combining to secure increased expenditure on the NHS under the present system (although at the expense of either taxation or else reduced expenditure on other public services), as discussed in Chapter 7.

Alternative Health Care Funding Systems

The worldwide explosion of health care expenditure during the past ten or fifteen years has been made possible by the increased willingness of governments to subsidise health care, and the increased willingness of individuals (or their employers) to join in risk-spreading health-insurance schemes. The triggers for these developments have been rising affluence, rising public concern for the care of the very poor and especially the elderly, and, in particular, the enormous rise in the costs of acute care relative to typical after-tax incomes of most citizens in most countries. Even in the (affluent) USA, almost the entire increase in health care spending has occurred because of the massive injection of government funds (Medicare, Medicaid etc.), together with the spread of employer-financed private health insurance.[5]

The structure and financing of health care delivery in developed countries spans a wide spectrum of arrangements. At one end is the USSR, with a wholly centralised health system. Near the other end is the USA, traditionally based on private medicine and a pluralistic delivery system, but being forced by rising medical costs and the pressure of public opinion to move further towards the central funding of a higher proportion of total health care costs, together with allied planning, monitoring and control systems. Most advanced European countries fall in between the USA and the USSR, with the UK (and to a lesser extent Sweden and Denmark) nearest to the USSR end of the spectrum (whilst still preserving the right of practice of private medicine), and most other advanced European countries placed in the middle of the spectrum.

We cannot here include a detailed description and assessment of the variety of arrangements in Europe (but see Maynard[6]). However, in summary, the mid-spectrum European countries differ from the UK in that (i) they do not have 'national' health systems, as the hospitals in particular may be owned by local authorities or charitable, religious or even private bodies; (ii) the funding of health care is indirect, typically through numerous health-insurance schemes (but with a variety of fallback arrangements for the needy and the aged); (iii) the system of primary care by general practitioners does not operate in the way or so fully as in the UK — so that much greater use often must be made of hospital out-patient services (or even in-patient services in some cases); (iv) there is more extensive use of 'fee for service' charging than in Britain, to discourage abuse and recover part of the cost; and (v) in some cases there is 'means testing' to determine an individual's degree of entitlement to full benefit from health insurance or other public health care funding or reimbursement schemes.

Our study of the available information does not lead us to envy the public health care delivery systems of other European countries. Their systems certainly appear to involve more complexity, and more waste of resources on bookkeeping and other non-productive paperwork, than in the UK. In Germany, France and Italy we can see no clear evidence of higher health care standards overall. In the Netherlands and Scandinavia there is evidence of higher health standards (and also of relatively much higher health care costs), but it is not clear to what degree the higher health standards (e.g. as regards mothers and infants) derive from the health care delivery system, relative to the effects of a generally higher standard of education, living standards and health consciousness among (especially) the less affluent proportions of their populations. In short, we see no clear evidence that these European (or any other developed) countries obtain better value for money from their health services than Britons receive from the NHS. Of course, that in itself does not prove that we could not improve our own NHS arrangements and performance at the existing level of expenditure, or that extra expenditure on the NHS (to bring spending nearer to international norms) would not prove worthwhile in respect of the incremental value for money obtained.

Possible Changes in Financing the NHS

We cannot blame others – especially persons working within the NHS– for proposing new financial and organisational arrangements that might make it easier to increase the total funding of the NHS – with a view to increasing the volume of health care delivery, the quality of equipment and other facilities, and the remuneration of NHS staff. Indeed, we would not reject an increase in funding provided it were demonstrated genuinely to benefit the public, and not solely or primarily to enhance the job satisfaction and remuneration of NHS staff. Whilst we have briefly considered arrangements in other countries, and have found no clear evidence of any more cost-effective arrangements than the UK already uses, nevertheless it may be helpful to consider specific suggestions that have been made for change within the NHS system of the UK. Let us consider the proposals put forward by the British Medical Association (BMA) in their *Evidence to the Royal Commission on the National Health Service*[7] (n.b. for ease of classification for comment, we have paraphrased the original proposals in the list below):

BMA Proposals	Our Comments
a. In place of health care financing based on allocation from central funds, there should be esta-	The quest for independent funding represents desires to (i) insulate the NHS from the political and economic policy of the Government, and (ii) facilitate possible

blished a separate Health Service Fund with independent sources of earmarked revenue.

growth in NHS spending greater or faster than might otherwise occur. Regarding (i) it must be noted that in fact UK Governments have provided the NHS with more stable funding, and more rapid growth than has been allowed to most other public services. Regarding (ii) the rates of charges levied into the proposed separate fund would of course remain subject to government decision, so that there could be no assurance of increased growth.

b. The revenue for the separate health fund would derive from three sources: (i) compulsory payments from all members of the population able to make provision for themselves; (ii) payments from the Government on behalf of all other members of the population; and (iii) payments made by the public for the use of specific services.

Item (i) is an expanded form of National Health Insurance (NHI): today's modest NHI contributions (included with National Insurance payroll deductions) contribute about eight per cent of NHS income. The proposed charges would increase health taxation levied from payroll taxes by a factor of perhaps six or eight; (ii) would be paid by the Government at the same rate on behalf of the elderly, disabled etc.; (iii) is discussed further below.

c. The compulsory payments under b. (i) above would be at a flat rate, collected from employed persons as a deduction from wages at source.

It is not clear why citizens should pay flat-rate taxes for health care when this is not expected as regards the funding of many other central government services. The proposal could be counter-productive in that there might be more popular resistance to increases in NHS flat-rate taxes than to increases in NHS funding supplied, as now, from the general pool of tax revenues.

d. Charges for specific services should be far more substantial than 2½ per cent of total

There is concern that new or increased charges might discourage or at least delay the demand for service from some persons most in need. There is also concern

NHS revenue presently obtained from this source.

over the cost of book-keeping etc. Charges would have to be expanded by a factor of at least ten, to achieve any major share in NHS funding.

e. Charges should include 'hotel charges' during hospitalisation (with arrangements to avoid hardship to old-age pensioners and the indigent), in recognition of the saving on patients' feeding and other domestic expenses while in hospital.

In many cases, patients' families may be worse off after income loss and the expenses of transport for hospital visiting etc. The costs of bookkeeping, collection and bad debts could be considerable. There is no assurance that governments would not simply deduct NHS revenues obtained by such charges, from the pool of government funding for the NHS (or from the rates of NHI approved by the Government). We recognise a moral view that patients should pay their keep in respect of non-medical care, but on balance we reject this proposal because of the disadvantages summarised above.

f. Charges for prescriptions should be continued, at rates to raise addditional funds.

Here the bookkeeping and bureaucracy of charging systems already exists. Perhaps these charges should either be abandoned, or else increased with inflation (as in the June 1979 Budget) and beyond to such a level as actively discourages frivolous requests for prescription (in respect of persons not exempt from charges on grounds of age or chronic condition).

g. Charges for consultations are not recommended (apparently because of time-consuming administration and waste of medical time).

A valid reason for rejecting consultation charges is that patients should not be discouraged from presenting themselves while their conditions are early and perhaps more easily curable. The argument based on avoiding time-consuming administration is valid, but no more and no less than with respect to other forms of charging suggested.

h. Fund-raising by voluntary schemes (e.g. lot-

We see no objections to such schemes, provided they contribute to the revenue

teries) are considered appropriate for raising finance for local projects.

i. The Government should continue to meet NHS requirements for capital expenditure: there could be a case for long-term loan-financing.

consequences of new developments, and not just the initial capital cost (e.g. of an extra operating theatre).

This is reasonable. The BMA presumably hopes by loan-financing to be able to expand the rate of capital investment (e.g. in new hospitals). Of course loans would have to be repaid, with interest: this and the extra running costs of the new hospitals would have to be met from revenue funds limited by RAWP criteria. We do not see this as a sensible and practicable proposition until such time as greater equalisation of resources is achieved, in accordance with national policy.

Our comments above explain why we reject most of the BMA proposals. To be fair, those proposals were made to the Royal Commission before RAWP and various more recent developments became fully known or understood. Even so, some of the BMA proposals still receive support in various quarters. The support, we think, derives partly from persons or organisations believing that health care should be paid for more fully and directly by each beneficiary of care (rather than from remote, progressive taxation); but mainly from persons or organisations who believe or hope that the enlargement of funding sources directly linked to the NHS will increase the total funding available to the NHS. The first reason for support depends primarily on moral judgements: there are two sides to the moral argument — we respect both sides and will not pursue the issue. The second reason is more relevant to this chapter: here we must express our personal doubt that the Government will behave otherwise than, first to decide upon the total NHS expenditure it considers justified in the light of economic circumstances and the needs of other public services, and then, secondly, to award its grant to the NHS after deducting from total allowable expenditure any revenue (other than charitable contributions) that the NHS may obtain from NHI or from charges for services rendered etc. If this is a correct judgement, then we conclude that time and energy should not be devoted to promoting major changes in the resources and methods of funding the NHS in isolation from any wider future review of the entire

UK fiscal and public-funding systems.

It is sometimes suggested that public understanding of the real costs of health care, and deterrence from unnecessary demands upon health care resources, could be assisted by requiring patients to pay for medical treatments (or at least hotel charges during hospitalisation), whilst allowing patients subsequently to claim refund of part or all of the charges paid. Here we have analogies to public (and private) health-insurance schemes operated in some other countries. Noting the cost of the administration and book-keeping for refund schemes in other countries, we doubt that equivalent costs would be justified in the UK by the educational benefit (or deterrence of unnecessary demands) that might result. In the case of poorer patients, considerable worry and temporary hardship might be caused needlessly.

Locally-based Health Care Funding

In place of altering the national system of NHS financing, it has been suggested that the latter should be retained but, in addition, AHAs or RHAs should be empowered (with due process, and within guidelines set down by the DHSS) to levy local service fees, rates or sales taxes so as to top up total funding to a level agreed with the local community as optimal for the scale and quality of health care (expenditure) that the local community desires and is willing to pay for.[8] Given that England has no regional government structure to match RHAs, in practice this line of thought forces one to consider its relevance at the level of the AHA (matching local-government entities). Two difficulties arise.

First, we believe that the AHA is based on too small a population to be cost-effective as a planning and management unit for self-sufficient resources in low-volume or high-technology clinical care. This view is held not only on grounds of cost, but also out of concern for the quality of care provided (which is likely to be of a lower standard if provided in many localities on a proliferated basis, at low volume with less-specialised and less-experienced staff). We suspect that much of the extra funds raised locally by AHAs, if the AHAs were allowed discretion in how to spend such funds, would be devoted to precisely these interesting and high-status clinical-specialty developments for which the AHA is not a suitable planning base. It is of course a matter of judgement where one draws the line in allocating different specialties as appropriate for development at area, sub-regional, regional or national levels. To illustrate that the problem is not unique to the UK, or directly derived from the UK's relatively low total spending on health care, it may be relevant to mention that in Sweden (affluent, with nearly the highest health care spending rate in the world; larger than Britain, with a population equal to two English RHAs) we are advised that it is now government policy that the highest technology specialties should be developed in only one centre (or, rarely, two centres). However, perhaps AHAs would use any locally raised funding only on cost-effective activities − such as community care and low-cost/high-volume specialties. That would resolve our first difficulty but, alas, not the next one. This is that it appears only logical that the more affluent local communities would be the most willing to support service, fees, rates, sales taxes etc., to assist the local AHA. Such assistance to upgrade AHAs' health care provision would appear to run directly counter to the functions of RAWP, and to the national policy objectives of equalising health care access and resources across the country.

Private Medicine

Controversy surrounds whether or not private medicine should be encouraged by public policy (e.g. by tax relief for private health insurance), and how closely it should be interlinked with the NHS (e.g. by sharing consultants and 'pay beds' with the NHS system). The supporters of private medicine argue that private medicine as an alternative to the state system constitutes an important personal liberty and right of the citizen; that private medicine can add to the total resources and health care available to the public; and that the comparison and competition between the NHS and private medicine can be beneficial to standards and progress.[9] We accept all these points in principle, but such acceptance does not of itself resolve the two main issues of controversy cited at the opening of this section.

The Scale of Private Medicine

There exist over 26,000 beds for non-acute care in private registered nursing homes.[10] These, together with other private residential facilities (largely for the elderly), provide the private counterpart to portions of NHS long-stay hospital facilities plus certain community care facilities. Indeed, these beds are widely used for elderly NHS patients where appropriate NHS facilities are not available.

Turning to primary care, the evidence is incomplete but it may be that two per cent is a likely maximum figure for the proportion of private general practitioner work done for private payment outside the NHS.[11] Owing apparently to public satisfaction with NHS family doctor services (as distinct from some other FPC services), private health insurance for general practitioner cover has not been popular or extensive in the UK. It does not appear that these services receive significant subsidy for private provision, nor that they involve controversy. There are controversies involving independent dental practitioners, but these relate mainly to the supply of dentists, the terms of their contracts and their 'fee for service' method of compensation from the NHS, and the division of labour between dental practitioners and the hospital dental staff. These controversies are rather specialised to dentistry and in general do not involve the main issues with which this section is concerned: we will not pursue them further.

It is in the field of acute hospital care that the presence of private medicine is strongest, and where the controversies especially arise. In private hospitals (and certain nursing homes) there are approximately 5,000 beds intended primarily for acute care.[12] This number of beds has risen during recent years, and it now exceeds the 2,500 or so beds still reserved in NHS hospitals for private use (known as 'pay beds' and discussed further below). Although the number of beds may seem large, their occupancy rate is lower than the NHS public beds – prompter admission and service is the essence of the appeal of private medicine – and the private health expenditure involved is probably less than three per cent of NHS expenditure on NHS acute services.

The total number of persons using private health services is unknown. The proportion of the population covered by private health insurance is under five per cent,[13] and the total users of private hospitals seem likely to be under seven per cent of the population, plus overseas residents who come to the UK especially for health care. It may appear strange that seven per cent of the population incur privately less than three per cent of the NHS acute care cost attributable to the remaining 93 per cent of the population. We cannot be precise on explaining the difference, but the primary cause is doubtless that the population able to purchase private health care (mainly through private health insurance) includes few elderly persons, and almost no one in the categories of the chronic sick or the socially deprived. In addition, emergency cases (e.g. road accidents or heart attacks) are generally dealt with under the NHS even where the patients have private health insurance. Lastly, the cover allowable under private health insurance, as also the available financial resources of private patients paying for care from their own funds, does have limits typically below the full cost of catastrophic conditions (such as cancer), so that in such cases private patients often must change over to NHS care when their private means are exhausted.

Although the proportion of NHS consultants holding full-time appointments in the NHS has tended to increase in recent years, it appears that approximately one-half of NHS consultants even now hold part-time NHS contracts.[14] Thus, approximately seven-eighths of total NHS consultants time is expended on NHS patients, whilst about one-eighth is unpaid (by the NHS) and is available for private medicine (however, one must note that the opportunities for private practice vary greatly as between different parts of the country, and as between different specialties). It thus appears that about twelve per cent of consultants' time (unpaid by the NHS) is available to deal with something over three per cent of total demand for acute care. It would therefore seem to be confirmed that consultants are able to give far more time to personal supervision of each private patient, than to the supervision of individual patients in the NHS. This does not signify that NHS patients lack medical supervision – the hierarchy of hospital doctors are present to provide medical supervision under the oversight of the consultant. Private patients may feel that they are receiving a higher standard of care, through the more intensive personal involvement of the consultant. Equally, we are advised, consultants appreciate the opportunity that private health care affords them to become more deeply involved in the cases of individual patients, because of the opportunity to manage cases in detail, and to observe and evaluate the effects of treatments. Many consultants would be delighted to be able to provide the same personal and close medical supervision through the NHS – it is not their fault that the NHS has too few consultants, and too many patients, for them to be able or allowed to provide the same degree of personal attention to individual NHS patients. In conclusion, we would

Pay Beds

Since the inception of the NHS, and following upon earlier precedents, the NHS has provided a fraction of its hospital beds to be available to private patients – i.e. patients paying a part-time NHS consultant a private fee for personally supervising their cases. In the early days these emphasise the diversity that exists. Many consultants do no private practice, and wish for none. Moreover, the demand and opportunity for any substantial amount of private practice varies greatly from specialty to specialty, and by locality (demand is less in Scotland, the North, and generally in poorer and rural areas).

pay beds were not especially controversial. Hospitals charged for the supporting services, but arguably the charges covered little more than the incremental costs of extra space, privacy and attention supplied to private patients. This seemed justifiable to the extent that private patients had paid their taxes etc. on the same bases as other citizens, and were therefore anyway entitled to full NHS cover for all health care facilities available up to the normal NHS standard of provision. By the early 1970s growing opposition from many workers in NHS hospitals to the provision of care to private patients, with support in Parliament, influenced the Government to decide to phase out pay beds (and thus private medicine) from NHS premises. This was embodied in the Health Services Act 1976, which established a Health Services Board charged to submit proposals for phasing out pay beds (and private out-patient facilities), to recommend arrangements for common waiting lists (as between NHS and private patients) for access to hospital beds, and to establish controls and monitoring over private hospital development.[15] At the time of writing these words it has just been announced (and here we have only press reports as sources) that the new Government proposes to abolish the Health Services Board, and to leave each individual Health Authority to negotiate over the future of its pay beds with its own local doctors and trade unions. This may or may not resolve the pay bed controversy in the short term, but we think that sooner or later controversy is bound to arise again at national level.

Arguably, the initiative to phase out pay beds was a mistake — at least so long as numerous NHS consultants hold part-time contracts and wish to engage in a limited amount of private practice. The NHS consultant who treats his private patients mainly within NHS hospitals is encouraged to concentrate his interest and loyalty within the NHS. Also, whilst treating pay bed patients he is still on NHS premises, and is available in case of emergencies involving NHS patients. In contrast, if he is forced to treat his private patients in private hospitals, the foregoing advantages are abandoned. Indeed, if the private hospital turns out to be newer, more cheerful, and manned by staff comparatively unaffected by the union problems, strikes and bureaucracy of the recent history of the NHS, then the consultant may well come to take greater interest in his private hospital links than in the NHS hospitals, to the detriment of the NHS and NHS patients.

The foregoing argument in favour of pay beds is — as it was at the time of the birth of the NHS — a pragmatic prescription. There is of course the counter-argument aired from time to time, that the British system of part-time consultants' appointments is bound to perpetuate delays and queues for non-urgent medical and (especially) surgical treatment – for the reason that it is these very delays and queues that create the main demand for private hospital treatment (and the resultant job interest and extra remuneration for part-time consultants). Certainly it appears to be a favourable promotion point for private health insurance – as well as the rational justification for business firms to pay for health insurance for their staffs – that private hospital care ensures early and convenient timing of hospital treatment, and thus minimum interference with employment. This ignores the fact that even for private patients, there are sometimes substantial delays in providing elective treatment (especially at teaching hospitals).

The right to choose a consultant and to have the personal attention of a consultant is another important promotional attraction of private health care. The third main promotional attraction, greater privacy, is paradoxical – (i) because largely equivalent privacy can often by obtained from the NHS, by request and payment for the underpublicised amenity beds; and (ii) because whilst privacy may be valued in anticipation as an important consolation during hospitalisation, there is a body of opinion that patients in large wards are generally happier (through the sense of community and the distractions of ongoing ward activity) than are patients in small wards or private rooms. Indeed this particular argument implicitly has been used by critics alleging massive waste of NHS funds on building hospitals more expensively than need be – partly to provide the greater privacy at that time deemed beneficial to patients, or at the least desired and valued by patients.[16] Of course, if an employer wishes an employee to continue some work during hospitalisation, then it is clear that privacy (and a telephone) would be considered essential.

The decision on whether or not to proceed with phasing out pay beds (so long as many NHS consultants hold part-time contracts) is a difficult one. We have mentioned above certain pragmatic arguments for retaining pay beds. Ending pay beds would remove about one-half per cent of the annual revenue of the acute-care sector of the NHS (without reducing costs by anything like the same amount[17]). This may not seem a large sum of revenue to lose, but it provides funds covering the costs of employing perhaps 2,000 NHS staff.

The debate also involves issues of equity and social policy. One may accept the existence of private medicine side by side with the NHS, yet nevertheless feel that it is inequitable that private medicine should be practised *inside* NHS premises, involving the privilege of earlier treat-

ment for private patients, and tying down NHS resources that otherwise (if, though only if, pay bed income was replaced by enlarged
government allocations) could be made available to NHS patients.
Degrees of feeling on this aspect of the debate are very personal, and we
must respect them. We think that, although pay bed charges have been
raised in the past decade by more than twice the rate of price increases
generally, full costs must demonstrably be covered, so that this economic point does not confuse the debate. (Charges can often exceed the
fees charged by private hospitals which may offer better accommodation and service, if not better care.)

The Government and Health Authorities have to decide policy on
pay beds, and in doing so have to consider not only the managerial and
moral arguments but also the practicality of a course of action. We
have mentioned some of the arguments in favour of retention of pay
beds, but this issue is contentious in principle, and retention has been
opposed by some NHS staff, who have indeed on occasion refused to
service pay beds. It is a matter of dispute and fine judgement whether
the Government should take a firm decision to impose (or negotiate)
this controversy centrally, or whether it would be better to leave
matters for local negotiation by individual Health Authorities.

Currently, in terms of the service provided nationally, pay beds
do not pose a significant issue in resource terms, though both Authorities and unions are becoming aware of the revenue lost to the NHS
itself, from the reduction of paybeds. Indeed in due course the further
growth of private hospitals, the high cost of pay beds, and delays in
treatment in some areas arising from the implementation of common
waiting lists may cause the demand for pay beds to wither naturally, in
which case they would be phased out gradually. But in London, pay
beds are an important matter and (especially if it becomes more difficult
to get certain treatments in NHS beds) private medicine (and pay beds)
may become increasingly important for the purposes both of raising
revenue and of compensating for shortages in NHS services.

As a footnote to this section, it may be relevant to mention one
factor we believe to be important, yet not widely known. We understand that consultants who are medical school professors, as well as
some other senior medical school consultant staff, are required by their
employment contracts to allow the fees earned for any private medical
work undertaken in pay beds to be paid over to the credit of medical
research funds in their respective medical schools. The aggregate of such
research income is not known, but it is believed that this use of pay

beds contributes a substantial sum towards the cost of medical research, and medical progress, in the UK.

Private Health Insurance

Private health insurance is heir to a tradition of providence and self-help through the pooling of health risks, that long pre-dates the NHS. This tradition contributed at least as much to the initial conceptualising and formulation of the NHS itself, as to the form of private health insurance (PHI) that has evolved since 1948, and has grown (from small beginnings) much faster than the NHS itself.[18] Whilst the resident population of the UK able and willing to pay directly from their pockets for private health care has fallen since 1948, the population able and willing (or assisted by their employers) to pay for at least their more routine acute care needs through the indirect and risk-spreading medium of PHI has risen from just over 0.1m shortly after the inception of the NHS, to some 2.5m subscribers and insured dependants, today.[19] The numbers above, and indeed our discussion throughout this section, refer to PHI provided by 'provident' institutions primarily to meet and reimburse the costs of private hospital treatment. There are of course other forms of insurance, mainly commercial, that provide cash payments in the event of illness, with a view perhaps more to covering loss of income, or consequential expenses, than to meeting private health charges for particular treatments: in this section we are not concerned with these latter forms of insurance.

Leaving aside the mainly London-based and often extremely expensive private health care provided for wealthy patients from overseas and from the remnant of the British rich, the main thrust for the development of private medicine in the UK centres around the principal PHI schemes, their managements, and the individual medical practitioners and institutions who support this development. Without PHI there probably could be no viable private health service in the UK, outside London. Any consideration of the merits and problems of private medicine (the care delivery side) must therefore give almost equal attention to PHI as the principal source for financing that care delivery. It has been argued often that private medicine is cost-efficient and can add extra funding and resources to the total supply of health care in the UK. This presupposes that private medicine can raise substantial funds − mainly through PHI − and that these funds are used to increase total medical resources and throughput, without significant detriment to the resources and funding of the NHS. We shall return to this important matter presently, but first it may be useful to summarise the experience of other countries that rely heavily upon PHI to finance their health care systems.

Health Insurance in Other Countries

A full discussion of the variety and tribulations of health insurance schemes in other countries, their problems and defects, and the remedies being sought, is not practicable here. The interested reader may wish to follow up our references, especially Maynard, if interest focuses in Europe.[20] The American scene is equally interesting, highly pluralistic in funding and delivery systems, and verging on the chaotic − but it is not easy to see what, practically speaking, could be usefully transferable from America to Britain.[21]

There are three main variant forms of health insurance: state health insurance (which we have earlier termed NHI); approved health insurance (AHI − local, voluntary or private bodies acting to collect and dispense health insurance funds, under greater or lesser supervision from Government): and private health insurance (PHI − largely independent of state supervision). In Europe and North America no country that we have noted has a system that matches NHI closely (although the issues are widely discussed). Perhaps the essential difficulty with NHI is that it cannot be a universal system − those in greatest need cannot afford to pay insurance. Health insurance developments in Canadian provinces come close to the NHI model (e.g. in Ontario), but clinicians are not fully integrated, nor has there been notable success in controlling the cost of health care.

What we have termed 'approved health insurance' (AHI) is the prevailing model in the European Community (see Maynard[22]). Many variations exist between countries not only in the degree of state supervision, but also in the degree to which AHI provides comprehensive (including catastrophic) health cover. In some countries participation in AHI sickness funds is compulsory for all (other than the elderly or chronically sick etc.), whereas in other countries participation is compulsory only below specified income levels. In the Netherlands a separate insurance fund for catastrophic cover is operated independently of their normal AHI schemes (whose cover is more comparable to PHI). In Denmark AHI was abandoned recently, in favour of a system of central government funding combined with local taxes. Germany has the largest number of separate funds: their number and the relative weakness of central control of health care spending owes much to traditions of regional autonomy. It has been suggested that these factors contribute to the high cost of German health care, by creating a bargaining situation in which the medical professions are in a strong position relative to the fragmented representation of health consumers' interests.

In most of the European countries the rates of contributions to AHI are set nationally and involve contributions from employers that are often larger than the contributions from employees. In this sense the European system is comparable to a social security tax (with which it is indeed combined in Italy) or to NHI. Where the approach diverges from NHI is in the plurality of the administering bodies, and in the degree of independence and variety of organisation of the health care delivery systems by which care is actually provided and charged. Typically, patients pay their own medical bills and then claim reimbursement from insurers (similar to the traditional arrangements under PHI). In most of the countries, insured patients are expected to pay a portion of medical bills, and/or a portion of prescription costs — partly to discourage excessive demands on services.

The European AHI systems are rooted in history: quite possibly public health care financing would have developed in a similar way in Britain if the NHS had not been founded in 1948 as a national entity involving central control of both funding and financial resource allocation. So far as we can see, there is no reason for the UK to revert to an AHI method of financing: it is certainly more costly to administer.

In the USA the past fifteen years have witnessed a decline in the proportion of health care paid for by individuals from their own resources. On the one hand, growth in medical spending has come from Federal Government programmes for the elderly (Medicare) and for the needy (Medicaid): much waste and fraud has been associated with these programmes, and increasingly the Federal Government has intervened with controls on spending and the pricing of health care services. There is a feeling that even the present arrangements are unsatisfactory, can be only transitional, and must lead on to some further form of deeper government intervention.[23]

The other source of funding for spending growth has been PHI. PHI is provided principally by two organisations closely linked to medical practitioners and hospital doctors (Blue Cross and Blue Shield), and by certain commercial insurance companies specialising in health insurance Unlike AHI generally in Europe, PHI is not a compulsory system. American PHI is available to individuals (e.g. the self-employed), but its main functioning is through group schemes linked to employment with the employer paying most or all of the cost Employer paid PHI often came into being in the USA as a fringe benefit negotiated by trade unions through collective bargaining. As in recent years American medical costs have escalated at a rate of increase several times greater than the rate of wage increases, it is reported that trade unions are greatly concerned at the way that increases in the cost of PHI pre-empt funds that otherwise might be bargained over with employers in respect of larger wage increases, or alternative fringe benefits.

Whilst the quality of American medical care provided under PHI is generally deemed to be good, medical reimbursement is on a 'fee for service' basis, and allegedly this leads to the provision of unnecessary or even undesirable services (e.g. excessive X-rays, or unwarranted elective surgery).[24] Most important, however, is that PHI cover has maximum annual limits, so that it does not provide adequately for catastrophic risk exposure — from which bankruptcy can follow, literally, in the USA. Nor does PHI provide a balanced and continuing programme of community care, or other care for the chronic sick.

PHI can cause additional difficulties (not necessarily restricted to the USA). PHI must be tailored to a balance between what the insured are willing to pay, and what is most essential to cover (i.e. to afford) within the amount paid. There are therefore various exclusions of cover relating to pre-existing conditions, which may on occasion trap the innocent, as well as reducing the general comprehensiveness of cover. There are also exclusions of certain new conditions (whether considered less important, or perhaps open to abuse), such as may cause doctors, believing in the need for care, to fabricate alternative conditions that qualify for treatment with reimbursement. This can cause alarm to patients, the carrying out of unnecessary diagnostic tests, and errors in medical records, statistics and research data. Lastly, whilst American PHI schemes have managed, at least nominally, to restrict the range of conditions covered, they have not managed to contain the explosion of treatment costs for the conditions covered. It appears that some PHI organisations have been insufficiently independent of the medical professions, that the PHI organisations collectively have been ineffective in bargaining with the medical professions to keep costs down, and that health care consumers — with imperfect knowledge and little organised bargaining power — have been ineffectual in preventing themselves from being exploited by the American medical professions.

Overall, PHI appears to have failed in the USA both as regards cost economy, and as regards the comprehensiveness of the health protection provided. Many alternative schemes are discussed in the USA, including alternatives with massive governmental involvement. The main development of immediate relevance to health insurance systems, however, is the Health Management Organisation (HMO). Whereas with conventional PHI one insures with a financial intermediary who reimburses costs on a 'fee for service' basis as charged by medical practitioners and hospitals that have no incentive for economy, the HMO situation is very different. Here one insures directly with a group of medical practitioners (the HMO), who guarantee out of the pool of insurance premiums received, to provide full health care services. The HMO subcontracts as necessary with outside specialists and hospitals etc. for the additional services needed by its patients. HMOs can compete for subscribers in respect of both their rate of charge, and the repute of the service they provide. Here the incentive is in general to minimise the cost of service delivery, both to attract new subscribers and to maximise the residual pool of subscription income – which supplies profits for distribution amongst the medical participants, as well as capital for improving the HMO's facilities.

The HMO seems an attractive concept, at least in the American context viewed as an alternative to the abuses of PHI systems in the USA. However, the HMO concept does not appear to be readily transferable to the UK. It relies on private practice and private hospitals as being the norm, and it needs the type of organisational environment found in the USA (but not in the UK), where no clear dichotomy exists between general practice and hospital practice, and where most doctors work as specialists both at the surgery/out-patient stage, and in the supervision of hospital treatment as well. Whilst the HMO system provides incentive to minimise waste and unnecessary treatment, and whilst so far the American HMOs are thought to have achieved a good standard of health care at a level of cost well below PHI (relative to the generally greater coverage provided), it is perhaps too early to be certain that the same results would obtain if HMOs covered the entire population, or that the temptation to possibly excessive economy in care provision will not lead to some lowering of health standards achieved in the long term.[25]

The Cost of PHI in the UK

Here we need to consider the total cost of PHI (and how far that cost may contribute to providing extra health resources), and also how the cost of PHI is divided up as among individuals, employers, consumers and taxpayers (and the possible effects of this division upon the nation's capacity alternatively to provide additional funding and resources to the NHS).

In 1977 the three PHI provident organisations that dominate the field received £86m in subscriptions, and paid out £71m in benefits to meet the larger part of insured patients' costs of £79m for the medical incidents claimed for benefit.[26] These sums are modest beside NHS spending, of course, and they represent less than three per cent of NHS expenditure on acute care in the year concerned. Thus five per cent of the nation's population were provided with acute care for under three per cent of total cost. Private medicine on this criterion would appear to be cost-efficient. However, persons insured under PHI are not a representative cross-section of the population: they are principally employed white-collar persons, their spouses and children. Moreover, private medicine does not in general provide the total spectrum of health care – especially the most intensive, expensive and prolonged treatments – as provided by the NHS. Serious accidents and other medical emergencies are probably more often dealt with by the NHS for the holders of PHI, than by private care. The NHS must provide large resources for the care of geriatric, mental, other chronic and terminal patients who do not hold PHI (and might never have been able to qualify for it), or the cost of whose care has already exceeded the maximum limits of cover specified for PHI.

For the foregoing (and other) reasons, it is clear that private medicine presently provides a much narrower range of health service than does the NHS. On the available published information we believe it to be impossible to compare the relative cost efficiency and effectiveness of private medicine and the NHS. Advocates of private medicine, and especially of private hospitals, argue that competition between the two systems would be healthful for both, inclusive of cost comparisons. It is our understanding, however, that the accounting methods and data are considered incompatible between the two systems, and we have not heard of any successful attempt to measure like with like so as to directly compare the two systems in a meaningful way.

One approach could be to attempt comparison of NHS pay bed charges for accommodation and other hospital services, as against private hospital charges. However, the case-mix in NHS pay beds is not representative of the mix of NHS acute care in general (for reasons explained previously), and it is impossible to determine with any degree of certainty what is the fair share of cost of the relatively small number of pay bed patients within the total cost structure (of paramedical and other back-up services etc.) of the NHS. The claim that private patients do not pay their full share of the cost (even though pay bed charges have risen by some 600 per cent in ten years, from admittedly modest rates) has become a prime resentment amongst those in the NHS who wish to see pay beds phased out completely from the NHS.

What effect has the expansion of PHI had upon the UK's stock of health resources — in particular, hospitals? Here the figures before us aggregate PHI expenditure with other private medical expenditure. Moreover, since the estimates published for 1976, there has been a reduction in pay beds, considerable expansion of the stock of private hospital acute beds, and an inflation in health care costs above the general rate of inflation. Thus, we are estimating in the dark in trying to assess the present situation. However, whereas in 1970 the private health expenditure was of equal magnitude as between NHS pay beds and private hospitals, by 1976 the expenditure at private hospitals was more than double that for private treatment within the NHS. By 1980 perhaps three to four times as much private medical expenditure will be in private hospitals, as in the NHS — and the amount of expenditure on mainly acute care in private hospitals may be of the order of £150m or more.

It is of course well known that the Nuffield Nursing Homes Trust, as well as other orgnisations, have been expanding their stock of private beds, especially since the future of NHS pay beds became doubtful.[27] Overall, it seems fair to conclude that the combined effects of the growth of PHI and the contraction of pay beds have resulted in an expansion of the stock of private hospital resources. The further expansion of PHI, combined with the ending of all or nearly all pay beds, should further expand the stock of private hospital resources. This could provide a net gain to the community, but only if the NHS did not lose resources consequentially. Based upon estimate, it appears that the NHS nationally (the local impact will differ widely) stands to lose about one-half per cent of its acute care budget if pay beds were completely phased out. This is nearly one year's growth money. Of course there would be a gain to NHS patients in terms of the release of beds, staff time and other resources, but inevitably NHS areas with many pay beds will suffer one or more difficult years of transition, unless the Government and DHSS are willing to allocate and earmark additional finance in compensation (which may be difficult to the extent that hospitals strong on pay beds and private medicine will often be in areas of above-average resource provision, which are anyway being asked to mark time in financial provision under RAWP).

But perhaps the key resource factor is staff, and especially nursing, paramedical and technical staff. In general, private hospitals do not train such staff, but instead recruit from the NHS. In many localities such staff are in short supply, and the ability of private hospitals to offer pay and working conditions marginally better than the nationally-agreed and inflexible NHS arrangements, poses a very real threat to the NHS. The growth of private hospitals does not provide a net gain to the stock of health-care resources.

Who Pays for PHI?

In the early years of PHI the subscribers were primarily separate individuals (together with their dependants). Subsequently, group schemes (which assist the pooling of risk and reduce administrative expenses) expanded, and increasingly private-sector employers became involved in financing group PHI for at least their managerial grades of staff. By 1972 employers were paying about 30 per cent of total PHI premiums. By 1977 this had risen to nearly 50 per cent, and there appears to be no reason to doubt that by 1982 employer-financing will provide any less than 60 to 70 per cent of total PHI subscription income.[28]

Employers may choose to pay part or all (increasingly it is all) the cost of group PHI for particular classes of employees — for the reasons that PHI can benefit the business by securing early and conveniently-timed medical attention for their staff, and/or that PHI is a fringe benefit that will help attract and hold good staff (bearing in mind also the benefits and attractions offered by alternative employers). Paying for PHI for staff thus appears in principle to be as legitimate a business expense as staff salaries and various other staff benefits and expenses. Accordingly, PHI premiums are normally allowable as a business expense that may be deducted from business income before determining business profits subject to corporation tax (except that eligibility for tax relief on new PHI schemes may be restricted at times of strict incomes policy). Yet this situation may give rise to two aspects of concern for equity — the one a paradox, and the other an anomaly. The paradox is that the Government should allow its tax revenues to be reduced in order that revenue that might go, *inter alia*, to the universalist NHS, is transferred to the credit of private medicine. The anomaly is that the opportunity to have employer-paid PHI is by and large restricted to private-sector employment. Public-sector employees are seldom eligible for employer-paid PHI — presumably on the grounds that public employers should not pay public money for a private service already provided at public expense by the NHS. Yet that is effectively what another arm of the public body — the Inland Revenue — allows to happen when tax relief is given to private employers in respect of PHI subscription costs!

We are not suggesting that employer-paid PHI subscriptions wholly escape taxation at the time of drafting these words (June 1979). Unlike certain other fringe benefits (e.g. company cars), the full cost of the benefit received in employer-paid PHI is added into the employee's taxable income, irrespective of the level of that income. While it will vary from company to company, and also as between individuals, in general the marginal rate of income tax of persons covered by PHI will typically be above the standard rate (now 30 per cent), yet well below the 52 per cent current rate of corporation tax. It follows that less tax is clawed back from employees, on average, than is being relieved on their employers – although the difference is not substantial.

At the present time the corporation tax and income tax systems treat employer-paid PHI in the same manner as salary or wage increases. Who ultimately pays for salary increases? Experience shows (barring temporary periods of freezes on prices, dividends, incomes etc.; and barring the experience of the minority of industrial firms suffering prolonged exchange rate and productivity disadvantages in respect of import/export competitiveness) that sooner or later the costs of salary increases (or fringe benefits in lieu) tend to get passed on to customers in the form of higher prices, at least to the extent that they exceed productivity gains. It is therefore arguable that under present arrangements the largest share of the cost of PHI is borne by the ultimate consumers of the products and services of the companies paying PHI subscriptions – and the majority of these consumers themselves do not have the benefit of PHI, do not have employers who will provide it for them, and are themselves totally reliant on the NHS. Is this equitable?

In Table 10.1 we include, for comparison, not only the situation that has prevailed under the tax laws of recent years, but also the distribution of cost that might occur if the recently elected Conservative Government were to implement its manifesto and Queen's Speech intimations of desire to assist private medicine (presumably through tax relief to employees and other individual subscribers to PHI). Also in Table 10.1 we include a third variant of taxation policy, disallowing corporation tax relief for PHI, such as would ensure more or less that the taxation system was not used as a vehicle to provide any subsidy to private medicine from the public purse.

Looking at the tax variant in the third column of Table 10.1, it might be thought too severe an imposition, unless it were applied, as a matter of policy, to discourage employer-paid PHI. One could of course disallow PHI for corporation tax, but in return remove the PHI pre-

Table 10.1: Who Pays for Private Health Insurance?

	Present tax system [1] %	Possible Tory tax change [2] %	Alter-native change [3] %
PHI Paid by Employers (Assuming Employers do not Increase Prices)			
Cost to employer (net of corporation tax relief)	48	48	100
Cost to employee (i.e. increase in his income tax) [4]	30	0	30
Reduction in govt. revenue (corp. tax net of income tax)	22	52	(30)
Total cost of PHI	100	100	100
PHI Paid by Individuals			
Reduction in govt. revenue (income tax relief to individual)	0	40	0
Net cost met from individual's own funds	100	60	100
Total cost of PHI	100	100	100

Notes:

1. The present tax system (normally) allows PHI as a business expense for relief to corporation tax, but treats it as a benefit in lieu of salary to the employee, subject to income tax.

2. It is assumed that tax changes contemplated by the Conservative Government would retain corporation tax relief for the employer, would relieve employees of income tax on the PHI premium, and would allow other individuals to deduct PHI they had personally paid for, from their incomes subject to income tax.

3. The alternative tax change would alter the present tax system only in respect of disallowing PHI as a business expense allowable for corporation tax relief (except in respect of employees working mainly overseas).

4. Throughout this table we assume an average marginal tax rate of 30 per cent for persons insured under PHI. In practice the rate will vary as between companies, depending how far down the salary hierarchy employer-paid PHI is provided. Looking to a future in which PHI promoters seek expanded coverage, 30 per cent may not be an unreasonably low average-marginal rate. When considering the cost implications for particular individuals, however, the tax relief (or burden) could be much divergent from the average, given marginal rates from 30 to 60 per cent at the time of writing. We assume 40 per cent as the likely marginal rate of tax for persons paying for their own PHI.

mium from being taxed as income to the individual insured employees. That, however, would actually encourage firms to provide PHI for their high-paid staff whose marginal rates of tax were above the rate of corporation tax.

Turning to the possible Tory Government tax change in the second column of Table 10.1, we see the opposite extreme to the severity of the third column. Tax revenues would be reduced by an average 30 per cent (but up to 60 per cent or any new maximum rate of income tax for high-income PHI subscribers) of PHI subscriptions paid for by insured individuals. As regards employer-paid PHI schemes, over half (on present rates of corporation tax) the cost of PHI would be paid for by tax reduction in the case where employers did not raise prices to recoup their expenditure on PHI (as might be the case where the promptness and convenient timing of private medical care really did materially benefit staff efficiency or productivity, or where total PHI payments were not large in amount, relative to profits). If prices were raised, the loss of tax revenue would be reduced as the price rise increased in scale, but the effective cost of PHI would then increasingly be imposed on consumers. Most consumers are taxpayers and also are present or potential clients of the NHS – they might prefer to pay more in taxes for an improved NHS sharing its benefits for everyone, than to pay more in prices to provide private health care for a minority.

The Total Cost of PHI

Extrapolating from published figures for 1977, and taking account of past trends, inflation, and estimated recent growth in the number of PHI subscriptions, it seems likely that total PHI subscription income will exceed £100m in 1979. As we have seen in the preceding pages and Table 10.1, it is impossible to be precise about who really pays for employer PHI schemes without knowing (and on this there is no data) how far employers recoup their PHI scheme payments by raising prices.

It seems likely, however, that whilst under the present taxation arrangements the situation is relatively 'neutral', and tax revenues are not significantly altered by the existence or growth of employer-paid PHI, yet nevertheless there is likely to be some consequential raising of prices, so that the consumer may pay a substantial portion of other persons' PHI (as well as the employees paying tax on PHI premiums at their marginal rates). However, even consumers paying higher prices can affect taxation revenues indirectly – to the extent that it may reduce their willingness and reasonable capacity to pay higher taxes to assist the NHS and other public services.

Suppose that employer-paid PHI were to grow to include about half the population. PHI on that scale could not be paid for without price increases to cover the cost, perhaps of one per cent or more. Here is an opportunity cost on a large scale. In lieu of encouraging PHI to expand, and tolerating the price rises it would cause, consider that alternatively one per cent could be added to the rate of VAT (or a one per cent sales tax earmarked for the NHS could be introduced) in order to assist the NHS to raise health care standards for the entire population.

Now let us consider the alternative we have hypothesised as possible Conservative policy to encourage the growth of PHI (column 2 in Table 10.1). In this case about 40 to 50 per cent of PHI costs would be financed by the taxpayers (i.e. by tax relief leading to reduced tax revenues), so long as prices are not raised because of PHI. Given the tax relief, price increases would be less than under the present tax system. But the tax relief would of itself stimulate faster growth in PHI, and given a sufficient scale of growth, then price rises would be needed to protect profit flows needed for dividends and reinvestment. It may not be unreasonable to suggest that a likely division of cost arising from the possible Conservative initiative would be perhaps 50 per cent paid for by the consumer (through price increases), 20 to 30 per cent paid for by reduced tax revenues, and the balance paid for out of employer profits (or perhaps productivity gains). At the present scale of PHI, that could mean, say £50m paid for by consumers, and £30m paid by reduction of tax revenues. Bear in mind that the £50m paid by the consumers to meet price increases, could alternatively have been paid in VAT, with the possibility of use in the NHS.

The above diversion from potential tax revenues is not an enormous sum. But suppose over a period of years PHI grew until it included nearly half the population. That would involve a tenfold growth in numbers, but total premiums paid might have to grow by a factor of 12 or even 15, for the reason that expansion on that scale would involve accepting a large number of persons with higher medical risk than are currently typical of the PHI population. In short, if such a stage of PHI expansion were ever attained, we would be dealing with a loss of tax revenues, together with higher prices (or lost taxable capacity), in excess of £1bn per annum.

Critics of the above argument may properly point out that if the Government had £1bn extra in tax revenues, it is most unlikely that under present conditions it would allocate all or even the major share of it to the NHS. They might argue that it is more important to inject extra money into health care, than to worry about whether the resources are injected into the NHS (notionally for equal sharing), or into private medicine (to be enjoyed by a minority who have been at least partially subsidised by other taxpayers and consumers). That is a matter of personal judgement. Our own viewpoint is that if the same energy, ability and money currently being thrown into promoting PHI and private medicine generally in the UK, were instead to be devoted to promoting the needs of the NHS to the public and to politicians, it could be possible to generate the political will to increase NHS resources considerably, even if not to the same degree that private medicine might attract resources if PHI did obtain greater tax relief. Certainly we would consider it inequitable to subsidise PHI and private medicine by increasing the tax relief available on PHI premiums – at the expense of reduced funds for the NHS and other public services.

Occupational Health Services

Michael Lee has calculated that in 1976 health care expenditure under PHI averaged under £29 per person insured, as compared to NHS spending of £117 on average for each member of the UK population.[29] Costs are probably rising more quickly in private medicine than in the NHS, owing to the capital costs of private hospital expansion, increased self-sufficiency and the higher proportion of consultants' costs in total costs compared to the NHS (n.b. the latter factor is relevant in the light of the ending of incomes policy). One may estimate that by 1979 costs per person insured under PHI have risen to about £50 per annum, as compared to about £160 per person per annum in the NHS.

These figures prove nothing as regards the possibility of better cost efficiency in private medicine. The main factors that explain the difference are probably as follows. PHI does not provide primary care, and in general it does not provide long-stay chronic or geriatric care. Typically it does not provide accident services, or full cover for emergencies and intensive care.

The bulk of the PHI population has the attributes of regular employment, above-average income and education etc., which correlate with better-than-average health. PHI may exclude poor health risks, or exclude treatment for pre-existing conditions. PHI has limits to maximum expenditure per person in any one year (most schemes currently appear to have limits of £10,000, £20,000 or £24,000 per annum: some schemes are index-linked for inflation). In some situations of catastrophic illness, PHI patients may have to revert to NHS care after PHI cover is exhausted. In short, the NHS provides wide-ranging care to all comers, whilst PHI provides a more limited range of care to a selected or self-selected subpopulation of below-average health care needs. The NHS has to try to provide the back-stop for all residual health care needs. This is a situation fairly unique to the UK.

In many European countries approved health insurance schemes have to provide a more comprehensive cover than does PHI in the UK: direct assistance from public health funding is often reserved largely for the elderly, the indigent and the chronic sick. The situation is similar in the USA, except that health insurance is not generally so comprehensive as in Europe, and catastrophic illness risk is a nightmare concern for many Americans.

The foregoing was not meant to imply criticism of PHI, or of private medicine more generally, in the UK. Rather it was meant to emphasise that the care provided through PHI is not a comprehensive health service, nor is it meant to be so. Indeed, the leading British provider of PHI, the British United Provident Association (BUPA), in its evidence to the Royal Commission in 1976, stated, 'In our view, the main role of independent medicine should be the cost effective treatment of the demand for elective medicine and surgery for the employed population.'[30] In other words, the role of PHI is mainly to provide prompt, conveniently timed 'elective' (i.e. non-emergency) treatment for employed persons (and often for their dependants). This role may be described as the provision of 'occupational health services'.

Elective medicine and surgery (e.g. hernias, replacements for arthritic joints etc.) is by its nature typically postponable. It is also the sector of health care where demand and the potential for health care interventions is potentially almost limitless — at least where such care is provided free of charge, as in the NHS. It is in elective care where waiting lists and queueing are a major problem. The practice of the NHS appears broadly to have been to work off waiting lists on the basis of degrees of medical need, inclusive of occupational risks affecting that need. Thus, a factory worker might face time off work, or else increased medical risk if he attempted to carry on at work without early treatment. The production manager of the same factory might suffer the same medical condition, yet be much less at physical risk in continuing at work, pending treatment. On these grounds the factory worker has the greater need and claim to early care and cure. This is a humane approach, but not necessarily compatible with occupational and economic logic. One absent factory worker can be covered by appropriate staffing, and be little missed from an occupational viewpoint, whereas the extended absence, or even the below-par working, of the factory manager may have serious occupational repercussions on the jobs of others, and on the performance and success of the factory as a whole.

Whilst one sympathises with the provision of treatment and priority according to each individual's medical needs and problems, it is clearly not an economically efficient way to determine priority for the treatment of elective conditions. To this extent, if PHI and private medicine can make good this gap in NHS provision, it may make a positive contribution to the UK economy. Perhaps it would be the ideal solution for the NHS to be expanded and improved so that it could cope with all realistic elective care needs quickly and efficiently for all comers, but that ideal is remote, and so in the intervening period PHI may usefully finance an occupational health service.

An occupational health service can have other useful features besides timely elective treatment for occupational convenience. For example, whilst the NHS provides health screening for certain occupations at risk — e.g. miners — it does not provide these services for the population at large (and especially, for white-collar workers). Private medicine linked to PHI can assist a wider provision of screening and preventive services than the NHS seems likely to afford, within its own priorities. Nor, of course, is all interest in PHI and private medicine centred narrowly on occupational objectives. We have heard of persons responsible for ill or crippled dependants, who obtain PHI to reduce the likelihood, in the event of themselves also becoming ill, of having to face delays in obtaining any treatment needed for them to resume the care of their dependants. It is a matter of regret that the NHS cannot be relied upon in such cases — or at the least, that the image of the NHS is such that some persons do not care, or dare, to rely upon it.

Finally, whilst we see a useful role for PHI and private medicine, and would wish to defend the individual's right of access to these services, we conclude that so long as it is public policy for the NHS to provide a high-grade universal health service accessible to all the people of Britain, then it will be unwise and inequitable to encourage the growth of PHI and private medicine by means, such as tax relief, that may actually reduce the resources available for the NHS.

Conclusions

In considering sources of funding for health care we are not primarily concerned with maximising the flow of *money* into health care. Rather we are concerned that any increased flow of money into health care resources should ensure that good value for money is supplied in return for the increase in funding (in which regard, better information, planning and control is needed, as discussed in other chapters); and that the money and resources are used to improve the NHS generally, in pursuit of its ideals since foundation — rather than to subsidise private medicine or encourage dual standards of care. Nevertheless, we do see a role for PHI in funding extended occupational health services (including health screening) — but short of providing a comprehensive 'alternative' health service. Even within the NHS, we are concerned at the risk of excessive localised self-sufficiency and proliferation of low-volume, high-cost services. To seek to fund a comprehensive private health system in parallel to the NHS would be the ultimate in waste of resources.

Whilst we may look with approval on the high standards of health care achieved (at high cost) in certain countries (e.g. the Netherlands and in Scandinavia); and whilst we have sympathy with those British clinicians who may look with envy at the greater supply of the latest facilities, and the greater financial freedom and recognition, available to them in certain other countries (e.g. the USA and Canada as well as several European countries), we believe that the NHS in Britain provides a relatively cost-efficient service.

If the British system does give better value for money in health care than most other countries obtain, we would ascribe that to the UK system of central government funding from general taxation, with allocations and budgets descending via regions and areas to the district and hospital levels. A contributory factor probably has been the UK reliance on salaries and capitation fees for remuneration, thus avoiding the temptation to overprovide services that occurs in countries remunerating medical staff on a 'fee for service' basis. We feel that pressure to expand the use of 'fee for service' medical remuneration in the UK should be strongly resisted by the Government.

We have considered other means of financing the NHS. Some alternatives would be directly or indirectly burdensome on the sick and the lowly paid. All the alternatives would involve increased paperwork, bureaucracy and expense in fund raising. On balance, we reject them in favour of the present system.

Although the evidence shows that successive governments have shielded the NHS from the effects of economic stop-go more than they have done for nearly all other public services, nevertheless the present arrangements can be criticised for providing inadequate growth. However, we conclude that rather than radically alter the mechanics of financing the NHS   which would not *necessarily* result in increased funding — what needs to be done is for the supporters of the NHS to make a much more effective and positive case to the public, and to the Government, to demonstrate (i) the need of the NHS, and (ii) that the NHS itself is doing its utmost to redeploy and optimise the use of its existing resources. This is a matter needing not just good public relations by the NHS, but improved accountability and sensitivity to the needs of the public, so that taxpayers may be educated to accept that the NHS is indeed worthy of increased support, priority and financial sacrifice from all of us who pay its bills.

Notes

1. *Public Expenditure on Health.* OECD Studies in Resource Allocation, no. 4 (OECD, Paris, 1977).

2. *Health Care, the Growing Dilemma*, 2nd edn (McKinsey and Co., New York, 1975), Ch. 2.

3. *Proposals for the Regulation of Hospital Costs* (American Enterprise Institute for Public Policy Research, Washington, 1978), Ch. 1 and especially p. 12; J.G. Cullis and P.A. West. *The Economics of Health, an Introduction* (Martin Robertson, Oxford, 1979), Ch. 11.

4. Ibid.

5. The four sources cited above are all relevant, and additionally may be cited: R.N. Rossett (ed.), *The Role of Health Insurance in the Health Services Sector* (National Bureau of Economic Research, New York, 1976); J.M. Rosser and H. E. Mossberg, *An Analysis of Health Care Delivery* (John Wiley, New York, 1977); M. Zubkoff (ed.), *Health: a Victim or Cause of Inflation* (Prodist, New York, 1976); M. Zubkoff *et al.* (eds.), *Hospital Cost Containment* (Prodist, New York, 1978).

6. Alan Maynard, *Health Care in the European Community* (Croom Helm, London, 1975). Also see OECD, *Public Expenditure* and McKinsey, *Health Care*.

7. British Medical Association (BMA), *Evidence to the Royal Commission on the National Health Service* (BMA, London, 1977), p. 24.

8. John Banham, 'Realizing the Promise of a National Health Service', *Evidence to the Royal Commission on the NHS* (London, 1978), pp. 3.11-3.12. 3.11-3.12.

9. BMA, *Royal Commission*, paras. 4.32-4.44 – although we do not accept all the points in these paragraphs.

10. The statistics here and in certain succeeding sections of this chapter are drawn, extrapolated or interpreted from two sources in particular: Michael Lee, *Private and National Health Services*, vol. XLIV, no. 578 (Policy Studies Institute, London, 1978); *UK Private Medical Care: Provident Schemes Statistics, 1977*, Report for the Department of Health and Social Security by Lee Donaldson Associates (London, 1978).

11. Lee, *Private and National Health Services*, p. 7 footnote.

12. Ibid., estimates based on data on pp. 14-15.

13. Ibid., estimates extrapolated from Table 2, p. 9. Also see Lee Donaldson Report.

14. Lee, *Private and National Health Services*, estimate based upon data on p. 16.

15. Ibid., Ch. 1, for detail of the background to the Health Services Act 1976.

16. Leslie Chapman, *Your Disobedient Servant* (Penguin, Harmondsworth, 1979), p. 201 ff., together with the BBC television programme based thereon.

17. Estimate, based on comparing NHS allocations with private medical costs reported in Lee, *Private and National Health Services*, p. 16 ff.

18. Ruth Levitt, *The Reorganised National Health Service*, 2nd edn (Croom Helm, London, 1977), pp. 11-16.

19. Lee, *Private and National Health Services*, extrapolated from Table 2, p. 9. Also see Lee Donaldson Report.

20. Maynard, *Health Care*.

21. See Rossett, *Health Insurance*: Rosser and Mossberg, *Health Care Delivery*; and American Enterprise Institute, *Proposals*.

22. Maynard, *Health Care*.

23. See American Enterprise Institute, *Proposals*; O.W. Anderson, 'Are National Health Services Systems Converging? Predictions from the United States', *Annals*, AAPSS, 434 (November 1977), pp. 24-38; 'Hospital Costs: Why the Federal Lid Won't Fit', *Citibank* (April 1979), p. 11 ff.

24. Radical Statistics Health Group, *In Defence of the NHS* (London, 1977), especially Ch. 1. Most American studies also comment on this problem.

25. Cullis and West, *Economics of Health*, pp. 271-2.

26. Lee Donaldson Report, Tables 7-9.

27. Lee, *Private and National Health Services*, p. 16.

28. Estimates based on Lee Donaldson Report, Table 7.

29. Lee, *Private and National Health Services*, p. 18.

30. British United Provident Association Ltd (BUPA), *Evidence to the Royal Commission on the National Health Service*, para. 5.5.

11 EFFECTIVENESS AND EFFICIENCY

Throughout this book we have emphasised that the NHS will never have enough resources to provide fully for those in need of health care. Given that funding of the NHS will always be inadequate to provide what is needed, it is absolutely crucial that the NHS makes the best use of the limited resources that it does receive. Wasteful expenditure quite properly arouses a sense of moral outrage because of the opportunities forgone to provide treatment for those who otherwise have to go without.

Although in Chapter 6 we recommended a strengthening of audit staffing and procedures in the NHS, this is, in the main, to ensure even greater confidence in probity. We see such measures as doing little to provide extra resources because there is negligible evidence of fraud, personal misuse of public resources, or other equivalent financial improprieties in the NHS. Little money is wasted by funds being misused in this straightforward legalistic way. But many in the NHS are concerned about resources being seemingly squandered every year in a 'spending spree' to get rid of unspent moneys remaining in budgetary allocations before the end of the financial year, at which time those moneys lapse. These exercises arouse strong passions, and although their magnitude and effects are probably exaggerated, their occurrence is serious in damaging the credibility of planning: people understandably wonder about the value of ordering priorities in planning when it seems that every year, in practice, priorities of claims are settled by ability to spend money quickly rather than by relative benefits to patients. We begin with a review of this spending spree not only because it is seen as one of the primary causes of waste in NHS financial management, but also because it illuminates other problems in budgetary control.[1]

The Spending Spree

Constraints at the End of the Financial Year

No one can measure precisely what is 'spending spree' expenditure as distinct from what would anyway have been purchased at the end of the year. Very likely, however, what is in question is a fraction of one per cent of the NHS budget. This sum could nevertheless be highly significant, especially for those authorities having to impose cuts which may be of the same order of magnitude as the money allegedly dissipated in such rushed expenditure. The primary cause of the rush to spend at the end of the year is popularly believed to be the financial constraints that cause unspent moneys to lapse. However, the Government has, for the NHS, exceptionally allowed limited virement and carry-forward to Health Authorities and Districts. But this flexibility has not generally been transmitted down to budget holders. Our own sample of enquiries within the NHS indicates that it is most unusual for budget holders to be allowed any automatic right of carry-forward at year end. That is, authorities and districts typically insist upon the (normally one per cent) revenue funds carry-forward – if indeed sufficient funds remain unspent – being earmarked for the authority or district as a whole, for new developments, contingency reserves, or other 'corporate' purposes. Thus, individual budget holders (i.e. functional managers) are not normally granted any carry-forward as of right, or with sufficient advance notice for this to influence their end-of-year spending commitments – and so the pressures to spend remain firmly upon their shoulders. The pressures are various, but they include the effect of the general conviction that the NHS is underfunded, so that it seems almost sinful to forgo any spending that is allowed (indirect services such as laundry and fuel costs expected).

As in other budget-managed organisations, there is also the constant concern that underspending will be taken as evidence of overprovision in a budget, so that the risk is increased of future budgets being cut back. End-of-year budget balances normally must be used only for 'non-recurrent' revenue spending. They cannot be used for 'recurrent' purposes that involve a continuing commitment in succeeding budget years – for the reason that such funding is not available, or has not been allocated to the use in question, in the next year's budget. Thus, for example, end-of-year surplus funds cannot be used to employ additional staff where such staff would normally have rights of continuing employment, and would thus become a charge upon recurrent revenue. Although financial constraints at the end of the year are commonly blamed for the spending spree, a second cause is the lateness in telling budget holders what their budgets actually are: in some cases three months of the financial year will have passed before the cash budget for that year is known. NHS authorities, management teams and finance officers are responsible for this – although one should recognise that they are constrained by the cumbrous NHS organisation structure, and its overelaborated tiers and requirements for consultation and consensus. The main factor here is the seemingly excessive delay involved in making successive reallocations down through regional, area, district and sector tiers until the level of front-line budget holders is reached. To be fair, it is not simply a matter of scaling earlier and provisional allocations of resources, as adjusted by the inflation-index assumptions of the final cash limits, when announced. The problem is that the cash limit will almost certainly result in a change in the volume of resources intended for the NHS from that planned at survey prices. This is because the allowance for inflation is likely to be different from that which takes place.

Whilst the Public Expenditure White Paper shows a steady (but limited) growth in real terms, translating these planned totals to cash allowances can mean irregular growth from year to year. When actual inflation may vary around the cash-limit allowance by a few percentage points, the switch from a generous cash limit to a stringent one can swamp the planned growth at constant prices. Health Authorities make their own judgements on whether the cash limit is generous or not, and re-examine their allocations accordingly. One reason for the need for lengthy consultations following the announcement of the cash limit is that NHS budgetary management focuses on the one per cent or so of growth money. We believe that this practice will have to change. But given this current preoccupation, if growth money appears to swell or to shrink by 50 or even 100 per cent as the result of final cash limit announcements, it should not cause surprise if each tier of the NHS feels obliged to review its incremental priorities before reallocating downwards. At RHA and AHA levels, moreover, final decisions must await scheduled meetings of the authorities – whose numerous part-time and unpaid members cannot be brought together at short notice for extraordinary meetings just to compensate for the Government's lateness in announcing cash limits. Even so, we believe that a greater sense of managerial urgency would allow the reallocation process, down to budget holders, to be expedited considerably.

We conclude this section with a general observation that the crucial influence on the spending spree is inflation, which lies at the root of several budgetary-management problems in the NHS, as in other public-service organisations. Inflation has made necessary the cash limits system, the late allocations to the NHS, and the necessity for further reviews and delay in reallocating cash limit funds downwards through the NHS. Inflation has also caused uncertainty for budget holders, causing the provident to hold back until the eleventh hour some reserve of spending, in case actual inflation accelerated beyond the provision built in to the cash limits. When actual inflation has fallen behind the provisions, then end-of-year balances have been large and have exacerbated the spending spree problem.

Budgetary Control

A second contributory factor to the year-end spending spree is lateness and inaccuracy in notifying budget holders what they have actually spent. This is part of a general problem of budgetary control, discussed also in Chapter 6. The general focus of budgetary control is to try to ensure that spending does not *exceed* budget allocations. This requires four factors for success: (i) frequent budget-spending reports, supplied promptly to budget holders; (ii) a low error rate, for the sake of credibility and discipline; (iii) a follow-up procedure whereby finance officers check on what has gone wrong, and advise budget holders on corrective action; and (iv) a fallback procedure whereby obdurate overspenders are subjected to disciplinary sanctions. At the time of our field research within the NHS — late 1977 and early 1978 — the NHS procedures were open to criticism on at least the first three of the above factors.

Budget-spending reports were supplied monthly but were not available typically until at least a month after the end of the month concerned. This is a delay at least twice as long as should occur. In mitigation, the delay can be explained partly by the inadequacy of NHS computerisation and the delays involved in areas and districts having to rely on RHA-based mainframe computers. Also, part of the delay can be explained by the present system being based on actual expenditure: what is important to the budget holder is what he has spent *plus* what he is committed to spend.

The second factor, a low error rate, is clearly related to the first. Attempting to reduce errors often appeared to be a cause of the delay in budgetary reports. The problems of reducing budgetary reporting errors, in turn, were due to the lack of adequate computerisation, lack of commitment accounting, and a shortage of trained staff, especially senior staff. This last point is of general importance. We believe that the level of management staffing in the NHS finance function is critically low; in industry it would not be tolerated; and indeed the level of spending on managerial and (non-medical) professional skill and expertise in the NHS more generally may be dangerously low. Specifically as regards finance staff, we feel that savings in costs of management by cutting and constraining staffing have been outweighed by a greater loss in the financial efficiency of the NHS.

The third factor, lack of adequate follow-up by finance staff to check on budget problems, and to explain these to budget holders and advise them on their problems, is again explicable by reference to the shortage of senior staff with relevant training in the NHS finance function. Perhaps the further point should be made that what the NHS needs in this regard, is not just a larger quota of senior finance posts, but a quota and salary structure of senior finance posts that will attract recruits from outside the NHS. Recruitment policy and the phrasing of job advertisements must also be orientated positively towards attracting finance staff (and also systems and computer specialists, economists, specialist auditors, planning specialists and other management scientists) from outside the NHS.

The problem is, in our opinion, that the NHS is so backward in developing finance and the other management disciplines that it simply does not have sufficient young people of ability, nor the appropriate training and experience in modern methods, to fill a majority of the needed senior finance and management appointments from internal candidates. This is not to decry the quality of most of the 'thin red line' of senior staff who now provide financial control and administration in the NHS, but the recruitment inflow of trainees and first-rate young staff does not seem large enough, nor the training opportunities adequate, to produce as large a crop of middle-grade financial managers as the NHS needs. At the extreme, we heard recently of one district — near London, where recruiting is hardest — that has only 25 per cent of professionally qualified staff in its posts of the level that should be filled by that calibre of staff. It is claimed that salaries are not competitive, and that currently the image of the NHS combined with the limited role for managerial discretion in NHS finance, make difficult the recruitment of able and experienced staff.

Lastly, as regards fallback sanctions for avoidable and unjustified overspending, these consist ultimately of the referral of any such case to the relevant team of officers, or, failing that, to the full Health Authority. In fact we ourselves have encountered no case that went so far as to involve dismissal or other heavy penalties. This could be construed to indicate either that financial discipline in the NHS is lax, or else that persuasion and more indirect sanctions applied through the financial system of resource provision generally suffice to secure acceptable budgetary behaviour. The true position seems likely to include a mixture of these two elements, but probably mainly the latter.

Budget Setting

End-of-year spending in the NHS represents but a small fraction of the total non-recurrent revenue budget, and the latter, in turn, is small beside the recurrent revenue budgets that cover pay, provisions, drugs and medical supplies, fuel and so forth. Any search for waste in NHS revenue spending must therefore concentrate upon the major routine spending of the NHS on its ongoing activities. Insofar as there is budgetary abuse in the NHS, we believe that this consists far more of slackness in the *setting of the original budgets*, than in any frequent failure to keep within budgets, once set. This is the problem, not unique to the NHS, that to the budget holder who holds most, or shouts most, the most shall be given. This is but another facet of the 'planning and budgeting for the increment' syndrome, that, whilst explicable and forgivable in the light of the past history of the NHS, becomes less and less tolerable with every passing year of increased pressure on slower-growing NHS resources. Quite separately, one may also challenge the scale and composition of new capital expenditure, especially on hospitals, as this tends to create and perpetuate new and higher levels of revenue spending even in cases where old hospitals are shut down and the total stock of beds does not noticeably. alter.[2]

It is generally recognised that no human organism or organisation exists without possessing at least a little fat. In financial control terms, such fat is termed 'budgetary slack': it is the margin of error, or padding, that every budget-holding manager seeks to have in his budget to cope with contingencies – without the uncertainty and worry of having to throw himself upon the mercy of finance officers or management teams in the event of emergencies, underestimation of need, or excessive inflation etc. It is the normal aim of finance officers in most organisations – notably but not exclusively business firms – to try to squeeze out as much budgetary slack as possible from managers' budgets.

In the business world, a 'blitz' on overheads is often initiated because of reduced profits and reduced volume of sales and workload. But firms frequently find it impossible to eliminate the slack by significant amounts (e.g. a ten per cent reduction in overheads). The attack on budgetary slack in the NHS is more difficult than for firms with reductions in volume and demand, because such reductions are rare in the NHS. Moreover, on average three-quarters of typical NHS budgets comprise wage and salary costs: given the continuity of workload pressure and the degree of job security typical of the public sector, it is not often possible to cut down significantly on this major element of cost. Even so, ideally the possibility of labour cost cutting (often feasible indirectly by not reappointing to vacancies when staff leave or retire) should be under constant review, together with the possibilities for other savings on purchased goods and services.

President Carter, when Governor of Georgia, was an early supporter of zero-base budgeting[3] – a shock-treatment method of challenging department heads to justify their budgetary requirements. Whilst there might appear to be a sense of unreality in budgetary reviews that appear to assume that a department or function needs no funds whatever, nevertheless this approach involves a toughness that in itself embodies a degree of virtue in the recognition of responsibility for the use of public funds. 'PAR' – Programme Analysis and Review – is a system with comparable features, introduced by the UK Government in 1970 for selective use, not as an annual procedure.

Resource allocation and control is provided at the operational level of the NHS by the system of 'functional budgets' described in Chapter 4. We carried out extensive enquiry as to the working of functional budgeting, in the course of our research for the Royal Commission.[4] In those authorities and districts not facing cuts or standstill of resources, the functional budgeting system operated on the basis of the previous year's spending being increased for the next year by the predicted index of expected inflation, with little or no dialogue occurring between the manager concerned and his management (or officer) team (or the finance officer, as representative of the team), to examine seriously whether or not any savings in real-resource expenditure might be feasible and desirable. What did receive scrutiny, mainly, were new developments (if any), the funding needed therefor, and the relative priority of these particular developments as opposed to other developments proposed by or on behalf of the other functions. Where authorities were being squeezed financially we found an attempt had been made to challenge existing budget levels by setting up *ad hoc* budgetary review committees. But the reductions made in operational budgets were not substantial.

Incentives

The alternative to the stick is the carrot. Managers (and indeed clinicians, insofar as they may be brought into sharing in the resource allocation decision-process, by specialty budgeting or otherwise) may be encouraged to take positive action in search of savings, by authorising them to transfer at least part of any planned savings achieved under one budget heading, to other budget uses and developments. During our field research we found variations in practice ranging from allowing no right of transfer or alternative use of planned savings by managers (on grounds that any and all savings should revert to the District or Authority's central pool of funds), to allowing 100 per cent transfer. However, a majority of authorities appeared to allow either 50 per cent or some reasonable and negotiated proportion of savings to be redeployed by managers. But typically such savings could only be used for non-recurrent revenue purposes, and would thus not necessarily have any resource redistribution effect in subsequent years. Moreover, these arrangements applied typically to resource redistribution *within* a single function (e.g. catering), whereas it would appear that the greatest need is for resource redistribution *between* functions, related to specific care-group priorities and programmes.[5]

Capital Expenditure

NHS spending on *replacement* plant, equipment and furnishings is in the main financed by revenue account funding, and, so far as we are aware, the amount of such annual expenditure is not readily determinable, although from discussions with NHS staff it appears that they think that the proportion of spending on replacement capital assets, as on the maintenance of existing capital assets, has been falling during recent years.

In general it is the cost only of new hospitals or other new premises, or major improvements or additions thereto – together with the initial plant, equipment, fittings and furnishings therein – which are classified as capital expenditure.[6] There have been allegations of waste of NHS capital expenditure in two respects. First, it has been noted that in recent years the NHS has acquired a number of hospitals that the relevant districts were unable to open, or to utilise fully, because of shortage of revenue funds. This does not necessarily reflect poor management. Hospitals designed at a time when NHS funding was growing considerably, and when the revenue cost consequences of enlarged and more sophisticated premises and facilities were almost automatically met by increased funding, were completed after the ending of Revenue Consequences of Capital Schemes (RCCS), and after the introduction of RAWP, which allocates revenue funds on a basis unrelated to the timing of opening new capital facilities. In some cases resistance from staff to the timely closure of old premises has tied down revenue funding that should have been used to open the new premises. In other cases the new premises and facilities have been so much larger, or so much more sophisticated, as to require a higher level of funding than the relevant health districts could immediately afford – at least as regards the opening and full use of all facilities.

Secondly, it has been argued that many recent hospitals were unnecessarily costly in design and construction. Leslie Chapman has made this point, claiming waste of at least £1,500m in the ten years ending 1977-8.[7] We are not clear how far the claim is deserved or could be fully substantiated, but from television coverage relating to the claim we infer that whilst part of the alleged extra cost may relate to insufficient use of standardised, low-cost construction, and/or to lack of firm management and consequential delays, a further part of the supposed waste relates to the extra cost of building hospitals with smaller wards, or wards otherwise designed to offer more privacy and space, instead of with basic, traditional Nightingale wards. The latter, large wards are not only cheaper to construct, but also are more economical of nursing time and running cost, because of compactness and the ease of ward visibility and supervision from a central point.

We are prepared to accept that substantial waste of capital moneys may have occurred, through underutilisation of standardised designs, lack of firm control on design and construction, and excessive sophistication in provision – yet we note, firstly that this judgement is the easier to make by hindsight (in the light of the only relatively recent lowering of expectations and aspirations regarding NHS growth and improvements); and secondly, that the evidence published is inadequate to prove that the waste was really likely to be anywhere near so great as the alleged £1,500m. Moreover, to the extent that some substantial part of the alleged waste appears to relate to more spacious and private ward designs (more expensive both in capital costs and in nursing running costs), there may be a paradox.

One of the important promotion arguments for private medicine and private health insurance is the greater privacy (and presumably spaciousness and other amenities more generally) that private care offers. Are the critics in effect saying, or at least implying that what is considered 'good' in private health care provision is 'waste' in public health care provision? If so, we cannot accept the implication that expenditure on amenity standards provided at above a 'least cost' utilitarian level for NHS patients, necessarily or properly should be described as waste! Is it the expectation that NHS amenity standards should be kept permanetly at a lower level than are provided in many other countries – including other countries (e.g. in Scandinavia and Canadian provinces) where hospital care is funded almost totally from public funds? We recognise that there is a body of opinion that a majority of NHS patients may be 'happier' or 'better adjusted' when in large Nightingale-type wards – by virtue of the greater fellowship and the distraction of the greater amount of visible activity and nursing presence. However, we doubt if there is conclusive evidence on this matter, or that generalisation may be meaningful. Public attitudes on this matter may well change (culturally) over time. The values set upon privacy may vary according to the type of illness, the seriousness of illness, the length of stay and the personal characteristics of patients (age, sex, class, regional cultural patterns etc).

Efficiency and Effectiveness in Supporting Services

When assessing performance and searching for possible waste, it is conventional to apply criteria both of efficiency and of effectiveness.[8] 'Efficiency' is the accomplishment of tasks with economy of resources. 'Effectiveness' is the attainment of objectives through tasks that are merely means to ends. NHS objectives involve curing, caring and improving health generally. Such generalised objectives can be refined in more precise terms for individual care groups, medical specialties and functional or service occupations. It is, however, extremely difficult to assess the efficiency and especially the effectiveness of services directly concerned with the provision of care, because the output of these services is so difficult to measure. We take this problem further in the next section. We consider here the supporting services (e.g. catering, laundry, supplies) where assessments of efficiency and effectiveness are more straightforward. Even here, however, the two criteria may be in conflict.

To take an apparently simple and non-controversial example, efficiency in catering is achieved by minimising the aggregate costs of provisioning and of food preparation and delivery, for a given standard of nutrition required. However, the fullest achievement of cost-minimising efficiency measures may not result in the highest degree of cost-effectiveness for the catering function, given that catering has objectives of contributing to the cure and care (and happiness) of patients (and staff), over and above physical subsistence. It is clearly not easy to assess what level of provisions and menu quality and variety, and form of service, will optimise the balance between the effectiveness objectives, and pure cost-efficiency. Indeed, strictly speaking, we would need also to be able to ascertain the opportunity cost (i.e. the relative benefit otherwise obtainable) of marginal changes in total catering expenditure, where such changes meant that more or less revenue funding was thereby left available for other health care uses.

In the case of catering, an attempt is made to balance the potentially conflicting aims of effectiveness and efficiency. The DHSS periodically issues guidelines as to provision costs for acute and other care groups. Our impression is that these guidelines are well above the minima necessary for adequate basic nutrition. Thus the DHSS has in effect uplifted minimum efficiency cost to include a premium of dietary quantity and/ or quality and variety, as an (effectiveness) contribution to care and cure. Health-care 'effectiveness' can include humane criteria as well as medical criteria. Each local health organisation is then left to organise its own level of desired quality in food preparation and delivery, with the guidelines to uphold standards, but also with the incentive to be efficient and minimise costs at the chosen level, in that savings in food preparation and delivery can be used in other health activities. The introduction into many hospitals of the advance selection of menu choices by patients, and the delivery of pre-served ('plated') meals in various sizes of servings, was presumably intended to assist efficiency (reduction of food waste) and effectiveness (release of nurses' time for other services to patients).

Here we must introduce a cautionary tale. During our field research − nearly two years ago − we heard only about the positive side of plated meals, as described above. More recently, we have heard it suggested that the impersonal plated meals that arrive on trolleys, just needing to be handed round, serve to destroy much of the valuable social atmosphere of meal-times for patients (especially long-stay patients) that was a feature of the previous system of serving and distribution of food delivered 'in bulk' to each ward. Even more important, it has been alleged that because 'plated' meals can be distributed by junior staff, or indeed by ambulatory patients, nurses need not supervise feeding, may not be present to see whether or not patients are eating all their food, and may become quite dislodged from one of their traditional roles of watching over the feeding and nutrition of patients. Malnutrition may occur.[9] We do not know how widespread or serious this problem may be, but its mere existence serves to illustrate how praiseworthy cost-efficiency initiatives may have unforeseen consequences that bring their ultimate cost-effectiveness into question.

Records are kept and studied of catering costs within the catering function (but not of the costs of food-serving on the ward). This consists of workload measurement and costing, and of course, the latter compared against the spending authorised in the catering function's budget. What is done for catering on workload measurement and costing, is done even more easily in functions such as laundry services, where effectiveness more nearly coincides with basic efficiency and where performance additionally may be directly compared with organisations outside the NHS.

Within catering, laundry and similar services, workload and costing measures may be sufficient to ensure reasonable efficiency — or at least an improving trend in efficiency — in using the stock of resources to hand. This need not suggest that the resources used have been acquired efficiently in the first place. In general, the costliest resource is labour. Wage and salary scales are agreed nationally. Depending on local demand-and-supply conditions for labour, NHS organisations may or may not be able to recruit and retain sufficient workers — or workers of sufficient quality. Certainly there is complaint from within the NHS — as also from within most other types of public-sector organisations — that central controls on wages and salaries, and on job gradings, result in an inability to compete with private-sector organisations in obtaining the highest quality of workforce. This varies from locality to locality, and it varies between occupations (according to the ease of transferability to other employment outside the NHS).

The second costliest resource is bought-in goods and services. Large private-sector firms act upon the belief that large savings can be made from bulk purchasing and firm contracts with regular suppliers. Within the NHS there still remains an element of waste, in that centralised bulk purchasing has not yet developed fully. The variety of NHS requirements is enormous, and sometimes items are needed urgently, in a sense not relevant to business firms. These factors, combined with traditions of localised ordering by the users of the item (rather than by 'professional' purchasing staff), and of ordering from local suppliers who have been helpful, have led to resentment and resistance to the full centralisation of purchasing in the NHS. Nevertheless, and in spite of complaints of delays and of incompetence of new purchasing staff (in the sense of lack of knowledge of specialised medical supplies and their suppliers), NHS authorities have been extending centralised purchasing and the holding of centralised stores. Centrally imposed controls on management costs, and on allowable gradings and salaries for attracting good-class purchasing and supplies-control staff, have almost certainly delayed progress to fully centralised and effective purchasing and stores, but nevertheless much progress has been made, and we believe the progress will continue.[10]

Budgeting For Medical Treatment

So far we have discussed efficiency and effectiveness only in non-medical activities. It will be remembered that clinicians are not budget holders. Currently, budgets are held only by the *providers* of the resources (including nursing and paramedical services) that are called up by clinicians as needed for the care of individual patients. Thus, budgets and the matching expenditure reports show us the cost of providing resources available for use in medical care, but they do not literally show us the costs of resources consumed. The number and cost of, e.g., bandages provided (i.e. purchased) in any given time period may not closely equal the number and cost of bandages actually consumed. Of course, over a longer time period, bandages purchased and consumed will match more closely, and the aggregate differences may be of significant interest only to accountants. What is more important is that because supplies are accounted for only to the budgets of providers, the records of costs relate only to the provision of goods and services, and not to the various uses and benefits for which they are consumed. Continuing the mundane example of bandages, the functional budget system provides a cost and a control upon total bandage purchasing, but it provides no measurement or control upon the costs of bandages used in casualty as compared to some other department, or as used or authorised by Doctor X as opposed to Surgeon Y.[11]

Bandages may be a trivial example. Enormously larger are the costs of nursing care. Here the budget (for the cost of provision) is held by a nursing officer, who must in practice respond to the demands of clinicians for care in each ward and theatre — within the limits of the total supply of nurses that can be provided by the budget and the wage structure allowed. Whilst the costs per ward or specialty can be recorded and monitored, the clinicians who call up nursing support are in no way budgeted, or held accountable for, the costs of the nursing support (or other services) supplied to them and 'consumed' in the care of their patients. Initiatives have begun to measure nursing workload and other (e.g. paramedical) services on the basis of consumption by individual wards, specialties or 'firms'. There are two points to make about these exercises. First, they have no official standing because clinicians do not work in any direct way against a budget: in the *course* of treatment they do not expect resource constaints to interfere, although these constraints may mean that treatment cannot begin, or may be of lower quality than they would ideally like. Once the arrangements for staffing, beds etc., have been agreed, clinicians expect freedom to make full use of those resources.

The second point is that costs are only one part of the data needed to make choices: benefits are crucial but cannot be quantified in a form to be set alongside costs. For example, open-heart surgery is bound to be more costly (per bed or per patient) than the correction of hernias.

A coronary intensive-care unit is bound to be more costly than a general medical ward partly filled with geriatric cases lacking alternative 'caring' accommodation. The extreme examples cited are almost sure to be true. Comparative costs on their own tell us little — although, even so, a trend of rising, or falling, *comparative* costs might give us clues as to relative performance and efficiency (possibly due to new drugs or procedures, and not necessarily to staff being overworked) being achieved in separate specialties. It is possible to assess effectiveness and efficiency of treatment within diagnostically homogeneous groups. But for planning purposes we have to make assessments across such groups.

Developments of Financial Information and Control Systems

Specialty costing is the collection and interpretation of the costs of activities specialty by specialty within the hospital.[12] Whereas functional budgeting offers aggregate costs classified by the departments providing goods or services, it offers no information on where and how the real resources are consumed, or their volume and costs used in or on behalf of the separate hospital specialties providing the ward and theatre-level contact with patients. Specialty costing seeks to remedy this information gap. The system is under development testing, with DHSS support.

Whereas specialty costing is essentially 'efficiency'-oriented, specialty budgeting is primarily 'effectiveness'-oriented (in the sense of our previous definitions of these two concepts). It appears to us that specialty budgeting is the more popular of these two approaches: certainly we know of several districts where specialty-budgeting development work is taking place.[13] Specialty budgeting involves the classification (i.e. across a matrix) of all those functional-budget expenditures that are reasonably traceable to, and responsive to, resource demands and consumption at the final stage, patient care, which is the province of clinicians. Such expenditures are traced, classified, and aggregated specialty by specialty. Whilst specialty costing is concerned with the detailed elements of cost (see below), specialty budgeting is more particularly concerned with the aggregates of those cost elements. Moreover, it is concerned with inviting clinicians to make expert judgements concerning the probable output value in health care achieved by particular aggregates (uses) of health care funds (budgets), as compared to alternative outputs that might be achieved by different permutations of expenditure. The new computerised Standard Accounting System (SAS) currently being developed will have the facility to process and report the relevant information for specialty costing and perhaps also for specialty budgeting. To fully implement SAS on these activities it will be necessary for authorities to provide improved computing resources, as well as some additional staffing for data collection (at ward level) and for data processing and interpretation. Similarly, it will be necessary for clinicians to give their moral support.

Using Specialty Budgeting and Specialty Costing in Deciding Resource Use

Given the complex nature of resource use by specialties, the appraisal of this resource use needs to be quite sophisticated. Specialty budgeting is one way of enabling clinicians to appreciate the resource implications of current practices and what is forgone in terms of new developments by not reducing existing expenditure. It does not of itself provide a framework for choice. The planning process should enable a more comprehensive approach to be taken. The vital link is between clinicians' decisions in hospitals, and planning by Health Authorities and Districts. In terms of the three-year rolling operational plan, the link between specialty costing and budgeting is fairly straightforward. Specialty costs give guidance on resource implications of new development. Clinicians can use specialty budgets to modify gradually their pattern of resource use. Operational plans can link to strategic planning by focusing on the changes identified as the outcome of the strategic review of future policies.

The problem remains of strategic planning for the development of, acute care. Linking specialty budgeting and costing to strategic planning may be best accomplished indirectly. In a previous chapter we suggested that in terms of the debate over priorities it might be most useful to disaggregate the acute care block not by specialties but in terms of client group — especially identifying treatments for the elderly. If this were the most fruitful approach then this would mean another classification of costs: a subdivision of specialty costs in terms of client groups to be aggregated, to produce costs by client group within acute care. This additional classification may be most appropriate for the political debate that seems necessary for the rationing of acute care. But the priorities that emerge from that debate would not appropriately be translated directly into constraints on resource use by clinicians. Rather, its purpose would be to give broad policy guidance to clinicians who have to make decisions on rationing. This is not to say, however, that there should not be monitoring of expenditure to see how aggregate clinical activity accords with the general policy decisions made through planning.

This problem is a difficult and delicate one which requires sensitive handling. We merely suggest an open-minded experimental approach, and caution is vital to avoid exacerbating what could easily be a deeply frustrating and alienating experience for clinicians in the future. The problem must be faced. Otherwise clinicians will face increasing conflict between expectations and demands from their patients, and what care can be provided with the available resources. They will have to deny treatment on other than purely clinical criteria, but will have no policy guidance as to what criteria should be applied. These other criteria are necessarily linked to the quality of life which results from medical treament and care. Because clinical judgements are vital in these assessments, the public at large cannot legislate on treatment. We need some way of mediating values on relative priorities, so that doctors can use these in rationing treatment. This occurs both at the level of treating the individual patient and when doctors fight for resources in Health Authorities' planning (in a role akin to that of a spending minister). Community Health Councils have a potentially vital role in this debate because they may be able to bring home to the consumer the link between what he would like to be given and what he is prepared to pay.

Notes

1. *Management of Financial Resources in the National Health Service*, Royal Commission on the National Health Service, Research Paper No. 2 (HMSO, 1978), pp. 121–7.

2. Leslie Chapman, *Your Disobedient Servant* (Penguin, Harmondsworth, 1979), p. 201 ff.

3. Peter A. Pyhrr, *Zero-Base Budgeting* (John Wiley, New York, 1973).

4. *Management of Financial Resources*. Also see I. Lapsley and M. J. Prowle, 'The Effectiveness of Functional Budgetary Control: an Empirical Investigation', *CIEBR* (University of Warwick, Coventry, 1978).

5. *Management of Financial Resources*, pp. 119–20.

6. A.J. Owen, 'Health Authority Capital Budgeting: the State of the Art in Theory and Practice', *CIEBR* (University of Warwick, Coventry, 1978). J. R. Perrin, 'Capital Maintenance and Allocation in the Health Service', *CIEBR* (University of Warwick, Coventry, 1978).

7. Chapman, *Disobedient Servant*.

8. Whilst we acknowledge the eminence of A. L. Cochrane's *Effectiveness and Efficiency* (Nuffield Provincial Hospitals Trust, London, 1972), we are using the terms 'effectiveness' and 'efficiency' in a different manner and context – more specific to management.

9. See papers in 'Developments in Clinical Nutrition' (a symposium at the Royal College of Physicians, London, 1979), where concern is expressed concerning the removal of nurses from close supervision of meals, and the risks of malnutrition, especially for cancer patients.

10. *Management of Financial Resources*, pp. 134–5.

11. Ibid., pp. 132–4.

12. Ibid., pp. 148–50. Also see C. C. Magee and R. J. Osmolski, 'A Comprehensive System of Management Information for Financial Planning, Decision Making and Control in the Hospital Service', *CIEBR* (University of Warwick, Coventry, 1978).

13. *Management of Financial Resources*, pp. 152–7.

12 IMPROVING ORGANISATION AND MANAGEMENT

The organisation structure and management processes of the NHS have been frequently and severely criticised since the 1974 reorganisation.[1] It is difficult to disentangle these criticisms from other problems unrelated to the reorganisation (for example, cuts in, and redistribution of, financial resources; and difficulties in industrial relations) and the need to adjust to the new structure, new style of management and new systems of planning and budgeting. In this chapter we review some of the criticisms that have been made, and the problems that we have identified. In a number of cases we suggest that as NHS staff become more familiar with their new tasks and gain mastery over them, a number of current problems will moderate. In other cases we suggest evolutionary changes that can be seen to follow adjustments that have already been made. We make no proposals for radical change: we are very well aware that the long-term benefits that such changes might bring could be vitiated by the problems of adapting to them.

The Increase in Management Costs

One of the problems of reorganisation is that, at a time when the growth in resources was being cut, the costs of management increased. This was to be expected with the introduction of new processes of planning, monitoring and co-ordinating at the three administrative levels, and the need to service extended networks of teams, committees and councils.[2] Indeed, between 1973 and 1975 the number of administrative, clerical and secretarial staff increased approximately 20 per cent. The extra money cost of the expansion of administration approximated to two per cent of the total NHS budget. However, even after the reorganisation, it has been claimed that the cost of administrative and other ancillary staff took up a smaller share of the budget than was the case in 1949.[3] Whether or not the increase in cost of management is justified depends not only on the alternative uses of the money for direct health care staff and equipment in the short run, but also in the long run it depends most importantly, first, on whether or not the reorganisation objectives of integration and co-ordination, and planning for change and redistribution, are themselves going to be a valuable benefit; and secondly on whether or not one concludes that the reorganisation and its extra management costs are achieving reasonable progress towards the objectives. We explore these points further in this chapter. However, since the reorganisation and the new systems are being used to alter past priorities of the NHS, it is not surprising that there has not been a consensus on the first of these points. Therefore, even if the reorganisation were being effective in terms of achieving its objectives it would still be criticised.

Criticism of high management costs should be assuaged by the fact that the DHSS claims to have reduced management posts in the NHS by some 2,700 during a period in 1976 and 1977 when other employment in the NHS was rising at a rate in excess of one per cent per annum.[4] In contrast, our own researches suggest that the NHS suffers from a shortage of trained and senior planners, management accountants, economists, systems and computer specialists, high-grade internal auditors and other management specialists.[5] It may be that management costs cannot be raised, if only for 'political' reasons, and that what is required is better systems, greater computerisation and a phased reduction in the numbers of lower-skilled clerical and administrative staff, to release funds for the appointment of extra staff with higher-grade managerial skills — so as to approach a level of management skills and staffing such as one might expect to find in large and progressive business corporations or nationalised industries. After all, the NHS is by far the largest 'nationalised industry'.[6]

Consensus Management

One of the important managerial principles set down in the Grey Book for the reorganised NHS is the principle of consensus decision-making.[7] This requires that officer teams and management teams should arrive at unanimous decisions — it is hoped — after thorough discussion of alternative points of view. Ideally, this approach would result in the fuller discussion of alternatives, in no single member of each team becoming more powerful than another, and in a collective commitment being reached to which all members of the team can give their loyalty. The criticisms are that the consensus approach extends the amount of time needed to reach decisions, and leaves extensive powers of veto in the hands of one or two intransigent members of a team, so that difficult decisions may never be fully resolved. Nevertheless, we cannot be certain that the overall effectiveness of NHS decision-making would be better if consensus were not required, and an alternative management style were followed. Certainly we cannot make fair comparisons at area and district level with pre-reorganisation NHS days — because both the scale and form of organisation, and the intended role of management, have been greatly altered, with the new emphasis on integration, planning and planned resource redistribution. Given the scale of altered circumstances, we do not have the evidence to prove that consensus management has failed, or should be abandoned. However, there does appear to be much evidence – if largely anecdotal – that the existing consensus management arrangements could be made to work more smoothly and swiftly.[8] Before we consider how this might be done we discuss the question of replacing consensus management with a chief executive.

Chief Executive

The NHS administrator, it may be argued, already has some of the powers and characteristics of a non-medical chief executive in the health service. He holds line-management responsibility for all the main ancillary functions other than finance and works. He has the responsibility additionally to co-ordinate the work of his team – which in practice means a duty to see that the other team members do carry out their work to some reasonable standard and time schedule. However, he has no authority over *how* the heads of other functions carry out their professional duties, nor does he hold any formal authority or responsibility over matters of clinical concern. Nor does the administrator necessarily even serve as chairman of his officer team or management team.

Unlike the Health Authorities, which have formally appointed chairmen with official duties, the organisation prescribed for officer teams and management teams carefully avoids creating formal chairmanships.[9] This is in the spirit of equality on the team, to facilitate consensus. In practice, some teams operate without a chairman, whilst others rotate an informal chairmanship: in all cases, however, it is the administrator's task to provide the secretarial servicing of the teams' agenda and flow of paperwork. In one district (and there could be other examples) we have been told that team members decided to persuade their colleague least enthusiastic about reorganisation, to take up the team chairmanship – as a way of stimulating his interest and commitment. That this risk was taken, in itself may illustrate the low level of 'blocking power' attributable to the informal team chairmanship role in NHS consensus management teams.

In large organisations where there are chief executives (or equivalents), this does not of itself remove the search for consensus. It is observable that the chairmen or chief executives of many kinds of bodies (including business firms) prefer to obtain consensus decisions if at all practicable. Again, in local authorities consensus management is widely followed, even though there is a titular chief executive, and in universities we have frequently observed chairmen and even vice-chancellors labour mightily to obtain consensus decisions on important issues – even when consensus is not formally required. It is only one aspect of management to exhibit speed in decision-making in the higher echelons of management. The more important and substantial matter is translating decisions into action. Without consensus of some kind from those who have to implement those decisions, managerial decisiveness may be to no avail.

The fundamental reason for consensus management in the NHS is that at the lowest administrative level (district or single-district area) the management team includes two clinicians. The practical alternative to this structure would seem to be a medical chief executive (it is doubtful if a non-medical chief executive would be acceptable to the medical and other professions). The first Cogwheel Report commented on this matter:

> For very many years the question of hospital administration has produced over-generalised and emotional debate often clouded by the question of whether or not the chief administrators should be medically qualified. A number of matters need reconsideration. What is meant by medical administration? How important should be the clinician's contribution to management? How can the clinician's participation in management be made more effective?[10]

These questions were addressed to the quite different organisation of the NHS of 1967. But their relevance remains. The critical contribution for clinicians to management in the future of the NHS lies in the rationing of acute care. It seems most appropriate to concentrate the scarce time of experienced clinicians who are prepared to take on administrative duties (either full-time or part-time) on this issue: it seems wasteful to train them in other administrative matters. One of the problems of the current structures of planning and organisation is that they are not designed so as to facilitate decision-making on the rationing of acute care. This makes the task of the hospital consultant on management teams a particularly difficult one. What is required is a better structure so that clinicians can reach consensus on rationing. Given such a structure, whatever style of management is chosen, the necessary decisions will be more easily resolved. Without it, changes in management style will have little effect.

It is relevant here to mention a recent proposal[11] that would assist current problems of medical administration. There is a serious shortage of community physicians in general, and of those who can take the lead in the planning of acute care in particular. The appointment of community physicians is rather curious in that those who worked in local authorities and knew little of hospital medicine are eligible for these posts, whereas hospital doctors are not eligible. This occurs even though 60 per cent of Health Authorities' expenditure is on acute care. It seems eminently sensible to create posts in medical administration for experienced consultants who would like to move across from treatment to play a major role in the planning of acute care.

The Weakness of Health Authorities

We have talked with a fair number of RHA and AHA members in the course of our researches. So far, not one authority member who had served on a regional health board or hospital management committee before reorganisation, has admitted to feeling as well informed or as well able to discharge his apparent responsibilities, as before the reorganisation. Here we must note that the responsibilities of authority members are potentially extremely onerous, involving corporate accountability and responsibility for the performance of their authorities in all matters not subject to clinical autonomy. The post-reorganisation weakness of Health Authorities (i.e. the governing bodies) may be attributed to the combination of several factors. First, the reorganisation involved such radical and extensive changes that the 'spare-time' and unpaid members of authorities were bound to need a lengthy period of re-education to master all the new complexities. Secondly, the Grey Book guidelines for reorganisation discouraged standing or specialist committees in authorities, thus reducing the opportunity for authority members to become deeply versed in particular aspects of knowledge concerning their own authority — e.g. finance and resource allocation. Thirdly, a side-effect of the adoption of consensus management in officer teams was that having once argued through an issue, and reached a consensus, officer teams were apparently often most unwilling to rehearse the alternative decision choices available to the authority, and instead preferred to submit to the authority only their single consensus recommendation for each decision, and the case supporting it. All three of these factors, taken together, might appear to throw in doubt the ability of each Health Authority properly to discharge its formal responsibilities to the RHA or the Secretary of State, as well as its implicit responsibilities to its own community. We will now examine the latter two factors in somewhat greater detail (the first factor is so straightforward as to need no elaboration).

One may infer that health authorities were discouraged from establishing committees of members (other than for appointments and for certain required duties under the Mental Health Act, etc.) because, first, the new authorities were to be a diverse mixture of individuals chosen from various backgrounds, and we believe it was thought that only the *full* authority could provide balanced and representative judgement (whereas committee substructures frequently turn out to be non-representative and self-perpetuating, in many kinds of organisations). Secondly, it may have been felt that the reorganisation's apparent emphasis upon upgrading the non-medical professions in the NHS (as represented through the officer teams), and its further emphasis upon consensus management by the officer teams, necessitated strengthening the role of the teams at the expense of the authorities, at least initially. Whatever the actual causes, the result seems clearly to have been an initial weakening of the power of authority members collectively, and a feeling of frustration and insecurity for individual authority members conscious of their nominally onerous, shared responsibilities. In the event, five years on from the reorganisation, we note that authorities are often forming *ad hoc* working parties or informal committees in order to enhance their abilities to have the facts and the understanding to cope with their officer teams and the various pressure groups that impinge upon them.

As regards the claim that in the first years after reorganisation officer teams often presented solely a formal consensus proposal to their authorities, and were reluctant to rehearse and debate alternatives, we can say only that we believe this was a mistaken extrapolation of the principle of consensus management; clearly, on any matters of substance for which health authorities corporately hold the authority and accountability for final decisions, they *must*, as of right, be informed and advised on the main alternatives, rather than be served up with a ready-packaged, single-choice, consensus decision proposal from their team of officers. A proposal can only be deemed optimal when it is supported by a reasoned case made in the light of the best feasible alternatives. Of course, it is understandable that teams of officers, new to working together in the consensus management aftermath of reorganisations, may often have been reluctant to reveal their own pre-consensus differences of opinions by presenting the arguments for alternative decisions to their authorities. But whilst understandable, it was also wrong. We are pleased to have heard that many officer teams have been persuaded to become more forthcoming to their authorities concerning the arguments for decision alternatives, and we consider it essential that this improvement of conduct should be adopted by all officer teams (and management teams, where relevant).

Remoteness and Delay in Decision-making

There remains one management problem related to 'consensus' that we have not yet considered. At the level of the individual clinician and the front-line manager, the complaint is frequently heard that since reorganisation it now takes far too long to obtain a clear-cut decision on important operational needs. Complainants appear to believe that delays are caused by (i) the reorganisation's drawing away authority from the hospital up to the sector, district or even area levels of functional officers, and (ii) the frequency with which functional officers insist upon referring problems to their teams — for a consensus viewpoint — before any firm decisions are announced. We accept that unreasonable delays almost certainly have occurred, and often, but we would argue that such delays have not been caused primarily by the consensus management principle, but rather by the abuse of that and other management principles embodied in the reorganisation.

Reasons for Delay

First, we believe that functional managers at all levels have not delegated as large a portion of the operational aspects of their authority to their operational subordinates as was intended by the Grey Book. Secondly, we believe that some managers and officers have shirked their proper responsibilities by referring problems excessively to their management teams, when the problems could have been resolved on the strength of their own authority, or by pooling their authority together with one or two other individual members of the management team. Thirdly, we feel that lower-level managers have too often sheltered within their own 'functions', have been reluctant to assume authority, and have missed opportunities to set up inter-functional co-ordinating machinery, however informal, so as to sort out problems at institution level, and, where relevant, to seek a consensus in their recommendations to their functional superiors in those cases where decisions formally must be taken at higher levels.

The first and the third of these criticisms interrelate to a point made in an earlier chapter: namely, that functional managers are not employing the budgetary system in a positive manner so as to delegate authority as well as accountability. In mitigation it must be recalled that functional budgeting down to the level of institutional or sector managers is only a development of one or two years' standing in some localities. Moreover, owing to the 1974 NHS reorganisation being so radical, relative to what preceded it – and owing to the large number of new managerial posts it created – it follows almost inevitably that a large proportion of NHS functional managers, especially at the sector and district levels, were not equipped by training or experience for the levels of *managerial* responsibility that they should have assumed in their new post-reorganisation appointments. Indeed many of these managers, such as nursing officers, may often have been selected more for their professional reputations and professional leadership, than for any proven skills in dealing with managerial systems such as budgets.

The Problem of Splintered Authority

At reorganisation, the hospital secretary who could order, coax or cajole a wide range of resources to meet clinicians' needs, was replaced by a sector administrator who was not necessarily even housed at the hospital unless it was a major hospital. Whereas the hospital secretary's post was often accepted as a career post in itself, under the reorganised structure the sector administrator's post is but a fairly junior rung on the career ladder of the administrator class of professional NHS officers. In general, the youngish sector administrator will not be able to attain the degree of local knowledge and authority held previously by the hospital secretary, given his comparatively shorter period of local service, and his likely orientation of loyalty to his profession within the NHS, rather than to his immediate physical location and workgroup. Indeed, the more able the sector administrator, the shorter his stay will probably be at sector level, before promotion! To be fair, this is not a problem unique to the NHS reorganisation: it is a phenomenon of modern management career-development structures that is widespread today throughout both the public and private sectors.

Aside from the altered career and status arrangements affecting new sector administrators, the changes made at reorganisation to reflect the upgrading and self-identity of other functional professional skill groups has served anyway to reduce the sector administrator's formal authority and capability to manage and deliver a comprehensive back-up service at hospital level. This is because many of the service functions, such as catering, laundry, maintenance etc., have had their physical organisation and/or their functional management centralised at district levels away from the direct contact and influence, let alone control, of the sector administrator. For example, many hospitals no longer have a handyman who can deal with a variety of simple problems such as leaky taps, when so instructed by the sector administrator (as nominal successor to the hospital secretary). Instead, because of (i) the increased relative cost of manual labour, (ii) the increased demarcation and professionalisation of most types of labour, and of the relevant specialist management as well, and (iii) the introduction of bonus payment schemes that require close specialist supervision to minimise abuse — it has come to pass, typically, that leaky taps can only be dealt with by a qualified plumber from the district works yard. The leak may not be dealt with until there are sufficient jobs in that hospital or at least in that direction from the works yard, as to make up an efficient bundle of tasks to assign to a plumber to undertake! Because of such constraints, we have heard of (even hot water) taps that have leaked for several weeks before being fixed. This is not to say that what happened was wrong or suboptimal, given present high costs of labour, but it clearly (i) is not necessarily the fault of the administrator, (ii) is not primarily caused by the reorganisation *per se*, but (iii) must be enormously irritating to the medical and other staff who have to work daily beside the leaky tap (during an era when staff are being exhorted to economise on resources!). What we are illustrating is a problem general to the present day social organisation and conduct of work — not a problem created by the particular form of the NHS reorganisation.

The issue that we have been illustrating is sometimes labelled 'splintered authority'. What may be done about it? Practically speaking, we cannot expect the clock of social evolution to run backwards to restore to the sector administrator the degree of personal authority and influence of the pre-reorganisation hospital secretary. However, one could conceive of a Sector Executive or Hospital Executive grade, with pay and career status comparable to a District Administrator, and with power to splice together and oversee the separate strands of splintered authority at the operational level. This would be recreating the hospital secretary's job, in effect, as a high level co-ordinator. He would acquire line or operational charge of most if not all service functions at the level of point of delivery, whilst leaving the sector and distrinct-level functional specialists to deal with the traditional functional and staff-specialist management duties of prescribing standards and methods (and recruitment, training and career progression), as distinct from the details of where and when service is delivered. This change would be substantial in scope, and for example, it would require the sector or hospital executive to be the principal budget holder for all the relevant services supplied to his organisation.

The above reform of the organisation would be fought by the various functional specialisms, because of the erosion of their own status and authority. If the will and political feasibility for creating sector or hospital executives do not exist, what else could be done? First, sector and hospital-level functional managers could be formally required to meet together as an operational-level management team, convened and co-ordinated by the sector administrator, and possibly with some degree of consensus required, as a method of re-combining splintered authority. Secondly, however, and this would be helpful in its own right even without the first element, sector-level managers need to use greater authority for independent decision-making within boundaries set up by their own budgets and by clear guidelines as to the acceptable range of service standards and practices, such as may be agreed or prescribed at district and area mangement levels in each functional specialism. Our own researches have suggested that managers in charge of functional activities at district levels often have failed to agree precise budgets with their sector and hospital-level subordinates, and have failed to delegate clear-cut authority to spend and manage within those budgets (as was intended by the Grey Bood proposals[12]).

Arguably it is the failure since reorganisation to co-ordinate the splintered authority of interrelated services, combined with inadequate delegation of budgets and decision authority more generally, that is the principal cause of the complaints of delays and failures in decision-making in the operational services. Where problems for decision have had to be referred up to higher functional levels because of inadequate authority delegated downwards, the higher functional levels have themselves apparently turned often to their management teams to gain the co-ordination necessary to make good the splintered authority. This has caused further delay, sometimes complicated by iterations of the proposed decisions until consensus has been obtained. Possibly much of this sad tale could be avoided in future by improved management within the existing Grey Book management arrangements. As managers become more adept at their roles in the post-reorganisation structure, and with clear budgets, clear delegation and firm pressure to use delegated authority from higher management levels, one may hope, and should be able to insist, that operational-level decisions become speedier and better, even where separate functions have to be co-ordinated with the decisions.

One Tier Too Many?

Almost every commentator who has assessed the NHS reorganisation, and also a number of major institutions whose submissions to the Royal Commission on the NHS have been made public, have expressed the view that there is one tier too many in the post-reorganisation structure of the NHS. Our own discussions with NHS staff frequently have elicited the same viewpoint. Additionally, politicians have picked up the argument and given it publicity. Where there is much smoke there may well be at least a little fire. But even if we do agree that there is a tier too many, the questions remains – which tier is least effective, least essential and most amenable to surgery?

It has been suggested that the district level of management should be relocated at the hospital level; that district management is superfluous and that its functions and staff should be divided partly downwards to the hospital level, and mainly upwards to integrate with the area level; that AHAs are bureaucratic and redundant and that their powers and staffs should be split amongst the health districts; that Health Regions are unnecessary and that their powers should be transferred to the AHAs; and that a commission for the health services should be formed to remove national health policy further from the political arena, taking over much of the present responsibilities of both the DHSS and possibly even the RHAs. We will consider each of these possibilities for further organisational 'reform' – however, we shall consider them not in the order listed above, but rather in order of increasing desirability, as related to our assessment criteria. In preamble, moreover, we should emphasise that major organisational change is disruptive; that the 1974 reorganisation was indeed massive and disruptive, so that managerial systems and behaviour even now have not totally adapted and achieved best possible performance under the new structure and the new rules of the game; and that any further major organisational changes within the near future should be undertaken only if there is high confidence of major benefits to be gained, as well as high confidence that the changes will be accepted and assimilated easily, by the NHS staff within the system, who must make the system work.

A National Heath Service Commission

The objective for establishing a National Health Service Commission would be to insulate the *funding* of the NHS from both party political pressures and short-run economic crises. This insulation could be provided either by favourable and guaranteed levels of financing from central funds, or by alternative funding arrangements independent of the annual division of the main pool of central government funds (e.g. by some combination of universal health insurance and point-of-service charging). One may reason that the health service is *de facto* a national-ised industry — indeed it is the largest single employer in the country — and that like other nationalised industries it should operate with a degree of management autonomy one degree removed from the short-run ebbs and flows of political controversy. Thus one might envisage the NHS being constituted as a public corporation, or at the least with a form of Health Service Commission at national level.

Nevertheless, the NHS is not like true nationalised industries because of the intensely personal services it provides (or has to refuse), and the social policy issues that result: this implies need for a form of organisa-tion different from other nationalised industries and more subject to detailed criticisms and guidance through responsible political processes. In practice there has, however, been little change between governments of the different parties in their funding of the NHS. Figure 7.1 shows that NHS expenditure has not been as adversely affected by recent economic crises as other major programmes of public expenditure. Moreover, one of the constant laments from chairmen of nationalised industries is that they are very much involved in short-term interven-tion by different governments. A nationalised industry sells its product or service into a market where it faces competition (or substitutes): its orientation to, and revenue financing from, a market gives it some degree of natural insulation from central government (although the Government at times intervenes in prices that can be charged, and in investment policy). Because these market factors do not apply to the NHS, an NHS Commission would effectively have little more autonomy from the political and economic judgement of the government of the day than does the present DHSS. Also, in our earlier discussion on financing the NHS, we reached the conclusion that (at least in the absence of genuine regional self-government in the UK, inclusive of independent powers of taxation) any change in the method of financing the NHS would be likely to increase the bureaucracy and the costliness of health care more than it would increase the quality and value of that care.

If the creation of an NHS Commission involved the abolition of RHAs and the division of their functions between the new Commission and the existing AHAs, we agree that there might be some saving on administrative cost — provided that most of the RHA functions were relocated at the Commission rather than at AHAs (whose large number would involve uneconomic replications of regional staff and services).

However, the administrative cost savings might be at the expense of greater central influence, if not outright direction, being imposed upon the NHS. We believe that the RHAs are in practice more insulated from the political changeability of central government than the DHSS can be, or than an NHS Commission could be (without independent funding). Moreover, the populations of most RHAs are quite substantial: they approximate to the populations of Norway or Switzerland; or an average American state; or any two average provinces of Canada. Such population bases would therefore seem large enough to provide a cost-effective framework for health service planning and management of all but the most rarefied of medical specialties and back-up services. We conclude that we see no present case to justify creating an NHS Commission.

Return Management to the Hospital Level

It is perfectly natural for clinicians and some others to wish to turn the calendar back to before the traumatic 1974 reorganisation. Nevertheless, it is necessary to remove the barriers that have segregated primary, hospital and community care. It is necessary to co-ordinate, and ultimately it is desirable to integrate these tripartite divisions of health care. Such co-ordination and integration will require that the effective power of health service management must reside at the level where primary, hospital and community care can be brought together 'in harness'. That rules out a return to autonomous management at the level of the hospital on its own, although (as we have argued previously) there are ways of making hospital-sector management both more efficient *and* more effective. And we pursue in the final section how the organisational structure we prefer can be better equipped to resolve the planning of hospital services.

Abolish Regions, Upgrade Areas

The abolition of RHAs, together with the redistribution of their functions downwards to AHAs, has been suggested. Although it does not appear to be a widely supported suggestion, nevertheless, its consideration may assist the development of our line of argument of desirable change in the organisation structure within the NHS. We have heard and read complaints that RHAs are too remote from local problems, too 'cosy' with the DHSS, too swollen with liaison and monitoring activities that largely duplicate work done at district and area levels, and too large (as regards the population and territory served) to provide the optimal base for planning health care provision.

Doubtless RHAs are somewhat 'remote' from local problems: equally, they are perhaps sufficiently distant as to be able to take a more objective viewpoint than can local personnel. However, in Britain — as in most other comparable countries — society is unwilling to provide the scale of resources that the medical professions and health-service managers would consider to be ideal. Therefore, inevitably at some level within the system there must be officials who have to say 'no' to requests for extra resources, or who ought to ask searching questions concerning the use of existing resources. If RHAs did not provide this function, then the DHSS itself (or an NHS Commission) would have to do so. Given that RHA staff are NHS personnel, not civil servants, and that most of the senior RHA staff have at some time served at subregional levels within the NHS, we think it probable that RHAs are in a position to provide a better-informed and more locally responsive service on resource allocation, monitoring and liaison generally, than the DHSS itself could provide if RHAs were abolished. There is, of course, the counter-argument that an expanded DHSS regional organisation could replace RHAs with possibly lower cost, greater independence from local pressures, and an ability to apply national policy more fully across all regions.

As regards the RHAs being too cosy with the DHSS, our own research does not support this. We see the RHAs and their staffs more typically as properly seeking to maintain a balanced stance as between national (DHSS) policy and the clamour of need and special pleading rising from the operational levels of the NHS. What is open to question (the circulation of formal DHSS circulars aside), is whether or not the DHSS has done enough to foster direct contact and communication with AHAs and their staff — so that DHSS views are known in an area in a direct and personal way. The problem may arise partly because the DHSS has relied too greatly upon RHAs as intermediaries in the process of communicating information along hierarchical tramlines. Now, whilst the RHAs have a primary role in strategic planning, capital expenditure, and long-term resource allocation, the dominant role (and the effective authority) for managing health care delivery is clearly based at the level of the AHAs and their districts — and we would urge the DHSS to improve the effectiveness of its direct contacts and communications with areas on operational matters.[13] We take up more generally the need for stronger links between the DHSS and the NHS in the final section.

The Grey Book prescribes an important role for RHAs in monitoring the performance of AHAs and their districts.[14] In the absence of a competitive market with the discipline thereby imposed on performance, alternative systems for monitoring and criticising performance must be provided. If the RHAs did not perform these functions, the DHSS would need to do so instead. We believe that the task is better done by RHAs, devolved and considerably sheltered from short-run political pressures by their corporate authority membership. When both RHAs and AHAs have adapted more fully to the reorganisation, RAWP and other altered arrangements, it may be possible to prune some overlap of administrative functions and to concentrate RHA attention on certain key planning and performance criteria, leaving AHAs greater discretion within the boundaries of the agreed criteria.

If the RHA tier were abolished and its key functions were centralised, we doubt that the same degree of devolved authority would, or should, be allowed by the DHSS to some 80 Health Areas (in England) as is allowed to the 14 RHAs. Indeed, as we have argued previously, there are a number of acute specialties, as well as specialised services, that would appear likely to lose economies of scale if AHAs (or indeed smaller local health authorities based on districts) were allowed to replace RHAs as the sole tier for strategic planning and resource allocation, and for co-ordination of specialties and specialised services.

Given our arguments, it follows that we reject the notion of abolishing RHAs, even though we would support the review, pruning and streamlining of their activities to what is essential to the distinctive RHA role. Moreover, bearing in mind the problems faced by small countries (e.g. Sweden and Denmark) seeking to provide a first-class yet economical health service, and also considering the considerable possibility that a good many acute specialties will in future benefit in both quality and economy from concentration in fewer centres than at present, we deem it quite possible that within a decade or so serious thought will be given to merging some adjoining RHAs so as to obtain larger and more economical bases for health resource planning and co-ordination.

Abolish Areas, Upgrade Districts

AHAs and their officers directly manage only a limited number of health care delivery activities. Instead the main role of AHAs would appear to be strategic planning, co-ordination and monitoring (leaving aside certain administrative and service activities that may (or may not) achieve optimal balance between local influence and economies of scale by being located at area level). To the extent that this simplified description is correct, it might appear that the main role of AHAs is largely to duplicate the role of RHAs at a lower level. Assuming duplication to be wasteful, and given our arguments that RHAs should not be abolished, it could appear logical that AHAs should be abolished. We argue against such abolition but equally we shall argue for a degree of transformation in the role and functions of (multi-district) AHAs.

Leaving aside the area-managed services, the bulk of health care resources at the operational level are administered by the District Management Teams (DMTs), who are accountable both jointly and individually to their AHA. The AHA's own team of officers (ATO) have a monitoring and co-ordinating role over the DMTs and over individual counterpart officers within the DMTs, but they do not have line-management authority over the Health District officers. Thus the ATO's formal function, area-managed services aside, would appear to have analogies to the functional staff departments located in the head-office organisation of many large business firms. This formal structure involves very delicately balanced powers and obligations, and it may all too easily lose its 'balance'. The ATO members, by force of personality and seniority, may come to dominate the DMT members. The ATO, by virtue of close linkage and influence with the AHA (i.e. the authority membership), may achieve tacit AHA support for ATO dominance over the DMT. The DMT, who are not now responsible for strategic planning as envisaged in the Grey Book and the original reorganisation initiatives, may adopt an assertive posture towards the AHA (and ATO), reacting against its diminished planning authority and in response to the pressures from below for resource provision in excess of the DMT's powers to plan for, let alone deliver, what is being demanded.

Perhaps the most popular argument adduced for abolishing AHAs and transferring their staffs and managerial powers to the district level is the argument that power should be brought down nearer to the operational level. Allied to this is the view that AHA staff duplicate part of the work of Health District staff, so that abolishing AHAs would allow a redistribution of staff and, in due course, a reduction to NHS administrative costs. As regards the latter argument, we believe that the claims of duplication of work (i.e. in planning, monitoring, record-keeping etc.) may have been overstated – and inasmuch as we have seen no evidence that NHS administrative costs are high by international standards, we believe this argument to be of secondary importance. Doubtless some savings can be made, or some administrative resources be redeployed to better effect, but this could happen whichever tier is eliminated, so it does not help us decide which tier to eliminate.

As for transferring powers to lower levels, we have already suggested the need for stronger functional delegation in association with control budgets, and the need for experiments with hospitals or sector executive posts, or other means of recombining splintered functional authority at the operational level. To achieve this does not require the abolition of areas, or of districts, although the abolition of either tier would serve to shorten lines of communication and consultation, and thus facilitate quicker decision-making. However, the essential point is that district management is *not* the operational level: it is the level immediately *above* the operational level, at which the separate strands of operations in primary, hospital and community care are intended somehow to be co-ordinated. A major argument for not abolishing the AHA is that it is an 'authority', not just a managerial unit. The authority membership, as a group of reasonable and responsible outsiders who are not local employees of the NHS, brings to the area level a degree of public accountability which justifies the area in possessing a degree of autonomy not practicable for district-level structures as presently conceived. It may be countered that districts could be upgraded by acquiring their own appointed authorities. This is true, but first it would involve a doubling of the number of authority membership posts, and considerable extra resultant expense and administrative servicing. Moreover, we have emphasised this point because we feel that some of the advocates of abolishing areas in favour of districts have made their choice precisely because they would prefer to see local health services more heavily influenced by health-service professionals and workers, without the present involvement of accountable lay authorities. This we would strongly resist. Nevertheless, districts could be converted into 'Health Authorities': our case for not doing so rests upon a further issue.

The decisive issue that leads us to reject any call to abolish AHAs is that of optimal self-sufficiency. Each Health District and Area comes under pressure from its staff and the public to become comprehensive and self-sufficient in health care resources. But it is the task of the overall administrative system to contain such enterprise within limits that provide – as nearly as one can assess it – an optimal balance between local self-sufficiency (and convenience to patients) on the one hand, and overall effectiveness and value for money on the other. It appears to us that current Health Districts, typically, are too small to provide an economical and efficient size of organisational unit for planning and delivering low-volume and/or high-technology acute care services. It is difficult at this stage to know how the NHS will resolve the problem of resource constraints and advances in medicine that involve very expensive treatments. If there is considerable development of such treatments, then optimising efficiency might necessitate removing so many specialties from smaller and non-teaching areas as to unreasonably dilute the ability of areas to plan comprehensive health care. Under such circumstances it would be worth considering the size of areas. However, we regard an explosive increase in the provision of high-cost specialties as most unlikely under current prospects. Therefore we feel that Health Areas, even including the smaller AHAs that are often organised as single-district areas, may well represent, for the foreseeable future, the optimal size of health care planning and co-ordinating units. They offer the additional advantage, given the present structure of local government, of being organised at the most useful level for effective planning contact with local authorities on community care and joint projects, not to mention direct liaison with Family Practitioner Committees.

Abolish Districts, Strengthen Areas

In the absence of an AHA, strong RHAs could curb excessive self-sufficiency in districts. We would, however, prefer to keep AHAs, but merging areas and districts. Districts would no longer be a separate and formal tier. There would be some increase in the number of areas.

Let us illustrate the seeming illogicality that can occur under present organisational arrangements. Leicestershire AHA is divided into three Health Districts.[15] All three districts radiate from Leicester. One district includes the local university medical school teaching hospital, with its natural claim and appeal as a centre for acute specialties. The second district includes, within Leicester, a substantial and long-established hospital in which a large volume of acute medical and surgical care procedures are provided. The third district also focuses upon Leicester but possesses no major acute hospital at Leicester. Yet, if our understanding of the situation is correct, that third district possesses the presumptive right (under the principles of the 1974 reorganisation) to establish its own District General Hospital (DGH): this is all the more likely to happen because Leicestershire, as well as the Trent region, of which it is a part, is below the national average in health care spending and resources, so that it may expect above-average growth in resources under RAWP principles.

It may be that, under the strict discipline of limited resources,

Leicestershire has been more efficient and successful than other localities in doing well with such resources. We understand that the bed occupancy rates and the average lengths of stay in hospital are quite favourable, by national comparisons. It follows that one must ask questions. Rhetorically, one may ask whether Leicestershire is under-provided, or whether much of the rest of the UK is overprovided? More practically, one may ask whether or not Leicestershire needs a third DGH — given that this third DGH might be built within a few miles of the other two DGHs, that it will draw upon many of the same senior consultants as the other DGHs, and that it may be presumed that the consultants concerned will prefer to concentrate their severe cases in one or two of the best-provided hospitals, rather than disperse their patients and fritter their own energies and travelling time amongst three separate DGHs?

This exposition is not set out as an argument against having three (or more) acute hospitals within Leicestershire. Rather, it is an argument against having three separate and nominally equal major hospitals within a few miles of each other in any urban area of that size. More urgently, it is an argument — with implications nationally and not just in Leicestershire — against the use of an NHS organisational structure which establishes an area management unit, plus three separate district management units with initial briefs to provide three separate but comprehensive hospitals, within so short a distance of each other. Quite possibly reason will prevail, with the third intended DGH being completed only as a smaller hospital with a more limited range of services. However, that would still leave the problem of three separate management units, one of which is heavy with resources as a Teaching District, and one of which has an average supply of resources, and the last of which may be short of acute care resources to provide balance in its provision of tripartite services. The question that must inevitably arise, is whether or not it is rational to allow one AHA and three separate district health-service management organisations to operate from a single provincial conurbation, where the total catchment-area population is less than a million?

What could be done in Leicestershire, as well as in other parts of England where somewhat similar problems arise, is to combine the Health Districts administratively with the AHA so as to form what is currently known as a single district area (SDA). The original use for the SDA was primarily to cover the case of a county (i.e. matching the criteria for an AHA) whose population did not justify the creation of more than one district. SDAs combine the status of an AHA (the essence of which is the appointed corporate authority membership, as well as a strategic planning role), with a management-team structure (the AMT, or Area Mangement Team) that includes the district feature of hospital consultant and general practitioner members. The DHSS will accept, and has accepted, mergers of Health Districts where such reform is locally welcomed and can be shown to improve efficiency.[16] Thus we are not here discussing a hypothetical reform, but rather one that is already viable and capable of extension.

Cornwall is an example of a county that has been an SDA since the reorganisation. It is larger in area than Leicestershire, although it has only about half the population. It has only one management team, which must be responsible for area planning and strategic activities, for area services and for the operational management co-ordination of local health resources. Below the officers of the AMT there are levels of supporting management at the SDA headquarters, as well as sector managers in the relevant functions. The essential difference in Cornwall is that important matters of general concern are dealt with by one team of officers — thus avoiding the problems of delay and confusion that may occur where separate teams of officers for the area as a whole, and for the district(s) concerned, are involved (in multi-district areas) in reaching their separate consensus decision as well as arguing their separate cases for AHA support.

The advantage of SDAs is that they combine strategic planning, monitoring etc., together with the role of co-ordinating and overseeing the delivery of operational health care resources. The AMT thus provides a closer analogy to the management team of executive directors in a typical large business, than do either the ATO or the DMT in NHS multi-district areas (MDAs).

Whereas Leicestershire might conceivably become an SDA in spite of its substantial population — on grounds of its having only one major urban centre and of the existing acute care and related service-planning and organisation apparently being largely structured radially around Leicester as a hub — this may be atypical. In many other MDAs factors of total population, its distribution, the number of major urban centres and the established pattern of acute care catchment areas (and hospital locations), may combine to suggest that many present MDAs should be subdivided into at least two SDAs.

From our own research we know that some members of AMTs in SDAs feel a concern that their role is made difficult by having to combine the district-level duties of being leader and protagonist for a particular service function, together with the wider area-level duties of planning, general monitoring and strategic consensus. Whilst one may sympathise for this concern for duality in managerial roles, we see the reconciliation of this tension as being precisely what higher-grade managers are selected and paid for, in most types of organisations.

AMT officer-members may have a justifiable concern, however, as regards not having been allowed sufficient senior supporting staff to provide the same calibre and quantity of oversight of the separable area-type and district-type management activities — necessitating the AMT members having to become too closely and personally involved in day-to-day management decisions. This arises where SDAs are deficient in senior and high-quality functional management staff at the next level below the AMT. It is these second-in-line officers who should be dealing with most of the day-to-day problems that arise in operational management. Indeed the DHSS should make funds available for increased senior staffing in SDAs. In particular, the SDAs that we have visited were, in our judgement, seriously short of high-grade management back-up for the area officers. This shortage of back-up seemed greatest in the fields of planning, information systems, management accounting, computerisation and industrial relations. Whilst the redistribution of lower-skilled staff (from the previous single AHA and the previous Health Districts being wound up) should fully suffice to staff the lower-grade posts in the new SDAs being created, in those fields just mentioned we see the need for outside recruitment and therefore for gradualism in conversion to SDAs. Gradual change is essential to avoid recurrence of the demoralisation that followed the 1974 reorganisation. (An additional reason for rejecting the abolition of AHAs and the upgrading of all existing districts is that the difficulty of providing sufficient high-grade posts (and skilled personnel to hold them) would be even greater and more costly given the larger number of districts.)

As regards the possible savings in management costs by conversion to SDAs, we see this as not arising from a reduction in senior management posts within the NHS, but rather as arising from a rationalisation and pooling of the clerical, administrative and other routines that, like separate premises, tend to accrete to any autonomous management organisation. In particular, financial and other information that needs separate checking, if not detailed handling, at both district and area levels in the present MDAs, could almost certainly be streamlined and more effectively computerised if processed only once — at area level. Indeed, any conversion from MDAs to SDAs should be accompanied by insistence from the DHSS that the lower-level administrative functions and premises of the former districts should be integrated and stream-lined as fully as possible. In return for such progress, the DHSS should be willing to accept selective expansion and strengthening of the higher-level management staffing of the new SDAs.

Resource Management with Two Tiers

Planning and Resource Allocation

We begin with a brief review of how planning and resource allocation might work in a NHS with only two tiers. Immediately, one of our major concerns about excessive self-sufficiency at district level is removed. Problems remain over decisions on patient flows across administrative boundaries, and on the rationing of acute care. The relevant systems for the resolution of these issues are the methods of the RAWP and planning. The RAWP methods are more reasonable when applied to larger administrative units, so again the change we recommend will improve targets as a guide for resource allocation. Nevertheless, decisions on cross-boundary flows will still be best informed through planning. Vesting strategic planning with both areas and regions has made the system extremely difficult to operate. It may be more efficacious to make regions solely responsible for strategic plans, and to make areas responsible for shorter-term plans – although the period might be extended to five or six years.

The Need for a Strong Regional Presence

We see the need for the RHA to exist as an independent and superior authority to its constituent AHAs. In a recent speech by Mr Patrick Jenkin (when still shadow Secretary of State for Social Services), it was proposed that RHAs should comprise consortia of AHAs: AHAs would elect members to this body.[17] We do not see this as a good way of providing the necessary regional presence for development of health services: as a creature of the AHAs, an RHA so constituted would tend to be relatively weak as a monitoring body, and weak in its ability to insist on vigorous regionwide resource co-ordination such as is needed, *inter alia,* to prevent the proliferation of small, highly expensive centres of medicine. Areas are an inappropriate level at which to vest the responsibility for new developments, because of the need to ration high-cost specialties.

Clinical Involvement

An important consequence of the change we propose arises from the fact that the Grey Book advocated the Health District as a focal point for health care planning and decision-making, because this was believed to be the largest administrative unit in which clinicians could be expected to be usefully involved in decision-making. But the mistake that was made was to conflate all clinical decision-making at district level. Whilst it may be the highest level at which clinicians can relate issues to their day-to-day work, this does not mean that it is the most appropriate level for all clinical decision-making. The Cogwheel system appeared to provide a flexible and effective framework for the management of clinical work within hospitals. The other committees designed to contribute to planning at district, area and regional level do not appear to have been successful, and the Area Medical Advisory Committee (AMAC) in MDAs appears often to have floundered. The removal of District Medical Committees will help reduce confusion and overlap. Cogwheel can continue in hospitals, whilst a committee with a quite different perspective will be required for the area: there would then be a clear dichotomy between the committees, not the current spectrum.

But a second problem of the AMAC has been the spread of interests which it has tried to represent. How can it both advise on the whole range of health services and yet also be representative enough to provide the necessary forum for the rationing of acute care, without being totally unwieldy? It is quite unreasonable to expect a body primarily designed to perform this co-ordinating function to be able to resolve the detail of any of its constituent parts.

The structures for clinical advice and decision-making need to be designed so that they can interact sensibly and efficiently. The care-group framework seems to provide a starting point. It is easy to see what is wrong with the current structure. We are naturally hesitant in proposing remedies for this complex problem. But given the logic of the argument, it seems the new SDAs might be most appropriately advised by medical committees structured in terms of care groups. They could then be seen to link to planning teams organised by care group. The problem remains that whilst the care-group approach provides a framework for deciding allocations across care groups it provides no guidance for decisions and choices to be made within acute care. The difficulty we can see is that rationing in planning terms may not be most usefully accomplished by dividing acute care into the specialty groups of the Cogwheel system: if we are to begin by focusing on the elderly, for example, it may be most appropriate to break down the acute care group in terms of types of patients. Thus, the clinical involvement in the planning of acute care may not be best achieved by an extension of the Cogwheel system. Here we are only speculating. We cannot make firm recommendations, since these must depend on how the acute care group is eventually disaggregated.

Improving Links between DHSS and NHS

Whilst we rejected the proposal for an NHS Commission we believe that there is scope for improvement in action at national level. The DHSS is part of central government. Its staff are civil servants, and few of them have first-hand experience of work inside the NHS. This detachment may assist objectivity but it involves the handicap of a lack of detailed contact and practical involvement with NHS management processes. Increased contact between DHSS and NHS staff, and a large increase in the interchange of staff, could assist the DHSS to provide a more useful managerial leadership to the NHS.

Moreover, it is arguable even if the DHSS provides effective co-ordination for the evolution of the NHS's own thinking on key issues. Certainly we feel that the DHSS does not provide the best feasible information services or guidance on the management activities carried out within, and essential to, the effective functioning of the NHS. It was for this reason that we previously recommended that the NHS — presumably through the medium of subscription contributions from RHAs and AHAs — should establish its own Health Services Information Centre to disseminate health-management research, 'intelligence', debate and possibly practical consultancy and field-training services.[18]

To illustrate the need, in our opinion there is a woeful lack of knowledge within the senior levels of the NHS as regards how problems of planning, funding and co-ordinating health care delivery are affecting other countries similar to the UK, and how they are attempting to solve these problems. Solutions may seldom be wholly transferable between countries, but at least their study should stimulate our own thinking.

Notes

1. Ruth Levitt, *The Reorganised National Health Service*, 2nd edn, (Croom Helm, London 1977), especially Chs. 10 and 11. *The Working of the National Health Service*, Royal Commission on the National Health Service, Research Paper No. 1 (HMSO, London 1978), especially, see Parts II and IV.

2. *Management of Financial Resources in the National Health Service*, Royal Commission on the NHS, Research Paper No. 2 (HMSO, London 1978), pp 142-3.

3. John Banham, 'Realizing the Promise of a National Health Service', *Evidence to the Royal Commission on the NHS* (London, 1977), p. 2.4. 2.4.

4. Department of Health and Social Security (DHSS), *Annual Report, 1977*, Cmnd 7394 (HMSO, London, 1978), para. 11.

5. *Management of Financial Resources*, p. 143.

6. *The British Health Care System* (Economic Models Ltd, London, 1976), section 4.

7. Levitt, *Reorganised NHS*, pp. 72-4.

8. *Working of the NHS*, p. 44 ff.

9. DHSS, *Management Arrangements for the Reorganised National Health Service* (the Grey Book), London, 1972), para. 1.27.

10. Ministry of Health, *First Report on the Joint Working Party on the Organisation of Medical Work in Hospitals* (HMSO, London, 1969), para. 28.

11. Grey Book, paras. 2.11 and 2.26.

12. Ibid., para. 3.40.

13. *Management of Financial Resources*, pp. 168-9.

14. Grey Book, para. 2.28.

15. Banham, 'Promise of the NHS', p. 29.

16. DHSS, *Annual Report, 1977*, para. 10.

17. Rt Hon. Patrick Jenkin, in speech delivered to the annual conference of the Association of Health Service Treasurers, 1979.

18. *Management of Financial Resources*, pp. 169-70.

13 CONCLUSIONS

We now draw together the strands of thought in the chapters of this book, and suggest some positive measures to specified groups of people — Health Departments, Members of Authorities, NHS officials, and the public as voter, taxpayer and potential patient.

We see the NHS, after its first 31 years, as a vital and massive development of public policy and administration, and of professional care. We consider that it must be retained, in a shape pretty close to the present. This is not to say that past changes have all been in the right direction, but that we must avoid unnecessary changes, after the disruptions of the last six years.

Nor do we think that all is well with the Service. However, despite widely publicised deficiencies and dislocations, and severe difficulties in some places, we do not see the situation as a widespread breakdown. But there are several long-term problems, still unsolved, which mean that the remarkable and basically successful experiment has now reached an extremely difficult stage. Our efforts to reach solutions are being watched in other countries which have been moving in our direction of greater government involvement in health care planning, financing and control; they are trying to find models which will avoid the problems the NHS has met.

The Shape of the Service

Central Responsibility and Financing

We would keep the basic structure of central ministerial control with reasonably defined, delegated powers and clinical autonomy. We would also keep the system of central financing, mainly from taxation. We reject (Chapter 10) the alternatives of a separate Health Insurance Fund, and of local financing of services, varying according to local decisions on the scale of expenditure. Locally variable financing would tend to undermine national objectives for the geographical equalisation of health care resources and access across Britain, embodied in the RAWP and other reports.

Private Care

We would preserve the right of individuals to purchase and to provide private medical care, and very probably this could sensibly include

the retention of pay beds in some hospitals, with indirect advantages
to the NHS itself; although in no case should private care be subsidised
by UK public finds. We think that Private Health Insurance should
be approached similarly: that personal tax relief should not be given
for premiums paid, and also that the effects and justification of the
present tax relief for group-insurance premiums should be closely reviewed (Chapter 10). Decisions in this would be for ministers and the
Inland Revenue.

Regions and Areas

We think that regions should remain, supervising and co-ordinating the
work of areas, but this would be in the context of a gradual move to
single-district areas (Chapter 12). In England this would mean that
planning focused on a wider geographical basis, and that the tendency
to uneconomic self-sufficiency would be reduced. Decision-making
would be improved and conflict within Area Health Authorities reduced,
and administration costs should fall somewhat.

Self-Sufficiency

Health Departments should give more guidance to authorities about
self-sufficiency. A more deliberate departure from district or area self-
sufficiency, with concentration of the more expensive and less commonly
used services in fewer places, may be good economy and also lead to
a higher medical quality of treatment. Inconvenience to relatives and
possible harm to patients are important factors; so are the advantages
of treating a patient for all conditions in the same building, but all
this has to be balanced against the cost of spreading very specialised
services too widely and thinly.

Health Authorities need to study the nature of cross-boundary flows
to specialised services, and decide which (in the light of national guidance)
it is right to continue, and where new local facilities should be built
up. These decisions could affect the distribution of capital and revenue
by Health Departments (Chapter 8).

Standards of Care to be Afforded

Guidance from departments about standards of acute care (where a
great amount of expenditure is concentrated) needs to make distinc-
tions within this very broad care group. Health Departments will need
to study intensively with authorities and clinicians how this can best be
done.

Some types of service are technically possible, as a result of research at home or overseas, but are not likely to fit within the resources on which the NHS will be able to call. Sometimes their original (perhaps expensive) developments may have to be forgone, even in 'centres of excellence': heart transplanting might be an example. More positively, we suggest that the DHSS should, in consultation, work out what long-term shape of the NHS can be afforded, so that regions can plan to develop services that will be needed and which will last. Guidance is particularly difficult because the results of innovation often cannot be foreseen, and the results of research (if mobilised and controlled with foresight) can save both lives and money.

London Teaching Hospitals

Central guidance of this kind is needed before the future of the London teaching hospitals (especially) can be decided, and before sensible decisions on funding can be taken. Meanwhile, the results of RAWP allocations are adversely affecting these great institutions piecemeal and through local decisions, and central decisions are needed as a matter of urgency.

Social and Clinical Priorities

There are also difficult and sensitive matters on the borders of social and clinical policy which need central guidance (and on which responsibility of a political nature needs to be borne). One is the allocation of resources to the sharply increasing elderly population, bearing in mind the high costs of combating the ageing process: problems of this kind arise also with the severest types of deformation and of injury.

Management

Within the cumbrous structure of tiers, and given the premiss of consensus management, we doubt if the costs of management are excessive. But management is not always as effective as it must become in this very large and complex industry, and we have several suggestions for developments over the next few years.

Role of Members of Authorities

To start at the top of an authority: the whole NHS structure depends on having an active and effective authority. This is particularly the case because its members are the only final co-ordinating and directing force within the region or area, given the absence of a chief executive in the official hierarchy. Their role has changed since the days of Hospital Boards and Management Committees, and they have now to govern an administrative machine in the first place, rather than a series of medical institutions. This means insisting on full service from officials without however putting wrong burdens on them: in particular, authority members should insist on knowing the alternatives to important proposals put to them. They should find whether good administration is being prevented by personal conflicts and inadequacies, and take action – because no one else may be in a position to do so (Chapter 12). They should see that the treasurer is much more than a bookkeeper – that he is brought into major building and planning work, and ensure that his department, and others, have the right types of staff ability for their future ranges of work – or establish why they cannot be recruited. They must be conscious of the genuine and recurrent difficulty of meshing-in clinical opinion (whether consultant or GP) to the administrative machinery, and try to establish whether advisory committees are working well and quickly: and similarly with other professional and staff difficulties, and consultation arrangements including CHCs (Chapter 11). We think that external recruitment and internal training should be improved if management is to be efficient: this may involve Health Departments as well as Authorities.

Delegation of Authority

Members and senior officials must, we suggest, give a lot of detailed attention to the delegation of authority, particularly to those administering functions and holding budgets at sector and hospital levels (Chapter 12). In conjunction with this, Health Departments should reconsider the general grading and career structure of hospital administrators: we feel that there must be a major drive to get enough delegation without losing co-ordination and central guidance, in order to get local decisions made quickly and without overloading teams at headquarters. This should aim to allow local officials to feel that they can do a good job of work with their professional and other colleagues, while properly representing the wider interests of their official or appointed superiors.

Medical Involvement with Management

We have left until last the most important point of management. This is the need for a radical overhaul of medical participation. The DHSS should review the working of Medical Advisory Committees. This also seems likely to require action by the DHSS, members of Health Authorities, administrative staff, and clinicians locally and through their national bodies (for example the BMA and the Royal Colleges). Clinicians have to ration their time in treating patients, and it is vital not to waste their time in committees. But the resource constraints within which they operate ought to be set with their full involvement. We suggest that the DHSS together with national medical bodies should review the medical advisory structure with the intention of providing broad guidance which is flexible enough to be adapted to local needs (as with the Cogwheel structure), and is consistent with progress in developing planning for the acute care group. Health Authorities then need to devise their own detailed structures to suit their doctors and local administrative arrangements.

But, more generally, each authority should consider immediately whether the clinical input into planning is being well managed – do officials and members feel they get responsible, adequate and prompt advice which helps with their strategic and operational plans? Members or officials might usefully talk to a few individual consultants and GPs (not just to representative committees) and ask whether they *feel* their views contribute to planning and to the taking of central decisions. This would also give a chance of asking whether paperwork already keeps doctors away from patients to an unreasonable extent.

Rationing of Resources and Services

When resources are less than desired, some form of rationing of services results, implicitly or explicitly. Members and senior officials need to work with professionals to see how this is working out in their services, and what guidance or action could be taken to minimise hardship, and particularly to use all existing resources to the best effect. This last point impinges on established habit and interests, but must not be dodged by perpetual 'incremental budgeting', as so often in the past. Guidance from departments on the future shape and standard of the service, suggested above, should help, but local analysis, persuasion and decision are what is most vital.

Specialty Budgeting

We view with interest and favour the experiments (Chapter 11) in 'specialty budgeting' – that is, giving hospital consultants or groups a budget within which to contain their expenditure and hence their services, while leaving clinical autonomy untouched. At present much hospital expenditure is the nominal responsibility of nurses, pharmacists etc., but the real influences come from clinical decisions outside any financial framework. Thus clinical decisions and behaviour must alter if significant resource reallocation is to be achieved. Health Departments will need to review results of these experiments and then develop a service-wide policy (Chapter 11).

A New Centre

Within the health service there seems to be room for a formal centre, supplementing the present good but scattered arrangements, where cross-disciplinary health-service management education and information services could be integrated: this would need action by Health Departments (Chapter 12).

Medical Education and Service Planning

Within medical education we feel that doctors must begin early on (though probably not as an extended formal part of their training) to think about the future shape of the Service – the balance between acute, long-stay and community work, and between advanced technological medicine and skilled application of present techniques: and to grasp and get ready to contribute to the perpetual problems of planning and rationing. Otherwise they are going to misdirect part of their training time and end up frustrated because medicine is not what they hoped. These themes may well connect with the studies in behavioural sciences and community medicine which have recently been developed. Some form of induction into the planning background would be valuable when doctors enter into senior stages in their careers. We commend these preliminary thoughts to professional bodies, to the universities and teaching hospitals concerned, and to the Departments of Health and of Education.

Clinicians in Planning Posts?

It may be that clinicians at a later stage in their careers may wish to move into posts which plan services for the community, on a part-time or full-time basis. We suggest that the DHSS (in the first place) should consider whether this is at present possible and should be encouraged (Chapter 9).

Salaries and Conditions

These affect recruitment and efficiency, as well as equity: but increases have to be paid for out of total taxes, which are not indefinitely elastic. We make no detailed recommendations.

Organising Information

What is Needed?

The information used for planning is deficient and must be improved if planning is to be taken seriously, as we think it sould be. This involves the flow of data internally, and also what Health Departments require the NHS to produce. We understand that DHSS are working in detail in this field.

Routine Returns

Information gathered by routine returns must be seen by the providers, whether clinicians or clerks, to have a real purpose. If they feel that it has not, much of it will remain unreliable, irrelevant, and little used. This is wasteful, ineffective and demoralising. Health Departments and officials of authorities should all examine the non-financial returns they call for, or have to provide, and check whether or not they are both useful and reliable. This exercise will not get done unless someone in full authority — the authority chairman? — puts his weight behind it.

New Developments

A very promising Standard Accounting System is being developed within the NHS. This will serve the needs of financial control (including commitment accounting, specialty costing and specialty budgeting if necessary), and of planning to some extent. The work needs to be given a strong impetus by DHSS, and decision taken there about the shape of information needed for central strategic planning (Chapters 5 and 9).

Analysis of Policy and Output

Strategic planning in the NHS is much more difficult than in many industrial firms, because the output from it is extremely varied. We do not seek automatic indicators independent of responsible policy aims: but as a longer-term objective we feel that analysis of policy and output assessment could be taken some way forward. Research has been done on the assessment of the outcome of medical intervention in particular diagnostic categories: the next question is how far there can be agreed assessments between such categories. Health Departments and individual officers and clinicians who are interested should encourage and collaborate in this long-term work, and see at what stage the results become useful in planning and in forming central policies on care or on allocation.

Voters, Patients and Taxpayers

What Does Your Service Cost?

Perhaps we may now directly address the reader who enjoys, suffers from, or pays for, the NHS. In thinking about the Service you must realise the high total cost in money and manpower (Chapter 2), and the very high cost of some operations, drugs and special nursing. Publicity by Health Departments of specimen figures would be startling and useful. Realise also that expenditure, after all the 'cuts', is still increasing quite apart from inflation, and that it takes a substantial slice out of people's incomes in the form of taxes they pay for it. You get good, though not maximum possible, value for money – and those who do not pay any tax get the benefits nevertheless.

Unwelcome Changes

To get the best value there have to be changes all the time. In particular, old hospitals may have to be closed to make way for new hospitals, or for new community-based forms of care. This disturbs habits and loyalties, but is the only way in which you will get better and up-to-date services in return for the resources people at large are ready to provide. (By the way, if you see that certain things are wrong or wasteful, don't just grumble – get in touch with your CHC.)

Do You Really Want a Better Health Service?

If, at a time of sickness, you feel you would willingly pay more for better service, realise that most people, for most of the time, are not calling on the Service. But they are still paying for it. Are you, and they, willing to pay a bit more for *other people's* sicknesses? That is the only way the money and staff can be provided to expand and improve the Service. Governments would soon move if people showed they cared enough to be willing to pay more. You may conclude that, on the whole, people are not really prepared to put their hands in their pockets in this way and to press politicians for higher spending and higher taxation. This book attempts to show how we can make the best of such a situation, by improving information and planning, and through better organisation and management control. Deciding on priorities and planning efficiently to achieve them will make the most of the devoted work of the people in the caring professions and of their technical and ancillary colleagues.

STATISTICAL APPENDIX

Table 1: (Tables and Notes for Figures 1.1 to 1.4) Health Expenditure and GDP — UK

	General government expenditure on NHS, £m		GDP at current market prices	NHS (1) GDPMP (3)
	Current prices	1975 prices	£m	%
	(1)	(2)	(3)	(4)
1949	(428)	(2380)	12.4	(3.4)
1950	(475)	(2620)	12.9	(3.7)
1951	494	2640	14.4	3.43
1952	506	2580	15.6	3.24
1953	531	2640	16.8	3.12
1954	546	2690	17.8	3.07
1955	587	2760	19.2	3.06
1956	641	2810	20.7	3.09
1957	693	2890	21.9	3.16
1958	735	2960	22.8	3.22
1959	795	3070	24.0	3.31
1960	867	3180	25.5	3.40
1961	937	3210	27.2	3.43
1962	977	3290	28.5	3.42
1963	1043	3350	30.3	3.44
1964	1138	3500	33.1	3.44
1965	1282	3690	35.6	3.60
1966	1407	3860	38.0	3.70
1967	1558	4080	40.1	3.89
1968	1693	4240	43.3	3.91
1969	1773	4170	46.4	3.82
1970	2024	4330	51.0	3.97
1971*	2299	4460	57.1	4.03 (4.15)
1972	2650	4646	63.1	4.21 (4.25)
1973	3013	4801	72.6	4.15
1974*	3934	4928	82.2	4.79 (4.75)

* See Notes about breaks in series.

	General government expenditure on NHS, £m		GDP at current market prices	NHS (3) GDPMP (1)
	Current prices	1975 prices	£m	%
1975	5299	5262	102.9	5.15 (5.13)
1976	6236	5355	122.6	5.09
1977	6879	5361	140.5	4.91
1978	7790	5469	160.6	4.85

Notes: Column 1 for later years comes from National Income Blue Books, Table 9.4, plus NHS capital consumption indicated by Table 9.2 (difference between total final expenditure and current expenditure on goods and services). Earlier years and provisional figure for 1978 from Central Statistical Office (CSO).

Columns 1 and 2 include the health services operated up to April 1974 by local authorities (but exclude, throughout, the personal social services). For the record (though there is no break in the series here quoted) the estimated expenditure in 1973 on local health services was: current expenditure on goods and services £185m (plus some capital consumption); capital £20m (1978 Blue Book, p. 130). They also include school health up to April 1974 (thereafter transferred to education programme and excluded from this series); the amount in 1973–4 was around £50m. Certain local authority health expenditure was transferred from April 1971 to personal social services and excluded from this series; the amount in 1971–2 was around £83m.

Column 2 excludes transfers (£20–30m in recent years – Blue Book, Table 9.4). Figures up to 1971 are from unpublished CSO data at 1970 prices, roughly converted to 1975 prices by multiplying by 2.15 (the ratio for 1967 and 1970 from a comparison of 1977 and 1978 Blue Books). Later figures from 1978 Blue Book, updated by CSO.

Column 3 comes from successive National Income Blue Books, updated by CSO.

Column 4: note the definition of this percentage. This is consistent with the basis for comparing public expenditure with GDP used by OECD and HM Treasury, but differs from that quoted in some other material* – see Note to Chapter 7. Note however that OECD compares health expenditure with trend GDP, not with the actual figures, and see notes to figure 7.3. The transfers of services to the health programme in April 1974 and out of it in April 1971 (see note to Cols. 1 and 2) mean

*Including Table E6 of the Royal Commission's Report (Cmnd 7615).

that the underlying rate of change in four calendar years is slightly different. Roughly adjusted figures are shown in brackets for these years.

Notes to Figure 1.3: This chart should be taken as approximate only. The sources are Cmnd 7439, Tables 1, 3, 6, 2.11 and 2.15; Cmnd. 7049, Table 5.11; and the National Income Blue Book, 1978. It has been assumed that GDP grows at two per cent from 1979–80 onwards.

Table 2: General Government Expenditure — UK (for Figure 1.4)

	On goods and services			Total
	£m	% of GDPMP	£m	% of GDPMP
	(1)	(2)	(3)	(4)
1949	2.50	20.2	4.45	35.9
1950	2.58	20.0	4.52	35.0
1951	3.31	23.0	5.37	37.3
1952	3.79	24.3	5.95	38.1
1953	3.97	23.6	6.16	36.7
1954	3.84	21.6	6.14	34.5
1955	3.92	20.4	6.46	33.6
1956	4.28	20.7	7.03	34.0
1957	4.45	20.3	7.62	34.8
1958	4.51	19.8	7.95	34.9
1959	4.70	19.6	8.43	35.1
1960	5.05	19.8	8.91	34.9
1961	5.47	20.1	9.73	35.8
1962	5.90	20.7	10.37	36.4
1963	6.24	20.6	10.95	36.1
1964	6.86	20.7	11.99	36.2
1965	7.48	21.0	13.31	37.4
1966	8.21	21.6	14.45	38.0
1967	9.18	22.9	16.67	41.6
1968	9.85	22.7	18.29	42.2
1969	10.26	22.2	18.99	40.9
1970	11.44	22.4	20.87	41.0
1971	12.83	22.5	23.15	40.5
1972	14.40	22.8	26.32	41.7
1973	17.03	23.4	30.50	42.0
1974	21.02	25.5	39.11	47.6
1975	28.2	27.1	51.5	50.0
1976	32.2	26.2	58.4	47.6
1977	34.2	24.2	62.0	44.1
1978	37.3	23.2	71.3	44.4

Source: *Economic Trends*, Annual Supplement, 1979, Table 135, updated, with GDP data from Table 1.

The Public Expenditure White Papers show, within Main Programme 11 (Health and Personal Social Services), figures for current, capital and total expenditure on 'Health'. These are on broadly the same basis as the totals for 'National Health Service' in National Income Blue Books, Table 9.4, for calendar years, the significant differences being (i) that Programme 11 shows Great Britain only, and (ii) that the White Paper figures exclude school health throughout but the Blue Book includes it up to April 1974: see notes to previous tables. The tables used are 2.11 from Cmnd 7439 (and Cmnd 7049, roughly revalued to 1978 survey prices), and 2.15 for Northern Ireland (with rough adjustment for social service expenditure and for capital expenditure).

The rounded figures are:

Table 3: Health Programmes and Capital Element – UK (for Figure 2.1)

Financial year	Health expenditure, 1978 survey prices		
	Total (£bn)	Capital (£bn)	% (2) $/(1)$
Actual expenditure	(1)	(2)	(3)
1972–3	6.2	0.67	10.8
1973–4	6.4	0.66	10.3
1974–5	6.5	0.54	8.3
1975–6	6.7	0.55	8.2
1976–7	6.8	0.52	7.7
1977–8	6.8	0.42	6.2
Part-actual 1978–9	7.1	0.46	6.5
Programmes			
1979–80	7.2	0.45	6.2
1980–81	7.3	0.46	6.3
1981–2	7.5	0.46	6.2
1982–3	7.6	0.46	6.1

Table 4: Principal Public Expenditure Programmes — UK (for Figures 7.1 and 7.2)

	Health and personal social services	Education science arts	Local environ-mental services and housing	Social security	Defence
Symbol on chart:	H	E	L	S	D
Actual expenditure				£bn at 1978 survey prices	
1970—1	6.5	7.4	6.4	10.6	7.2
1971—2	6.7	7.9	6.2	11.3	7.3
1972—3	7.2	8.4	6.3	11.9	7.1
1973—4	7.6	9.0	7.6	11.9	7.0
1974—5	7.8	9.0	9.6	12.7	6.8
1975—6	8.1	9.2	9.0	13.8	7.1
1976—7	8.2	9.2	8.7	14.2	7.0
1977—8	8.2	8.8	8.0	14.7	6.8
Part-actual					
1978—9	8.5	9.0	8.3	15.8	6.9
Programmes					
1979—80	8.7	9.1	8.6	16.3	7.2
1980—81	8.8	9.2	8.9	16.6	7.4
1981—2	9.0	9.2	9.1	16.8	7.4
1982—3	9.2	9.2	9.2	17.1	7.4
				Percentage changes from previous year	
1971—2	4.0	7.2	-3.0	6.2	1.3
1972—3	6.8	7.0	1.0	5.6	-2.1
1973—4	5.2	5.4	20.1	0.1	-1.3
1974—5	2.4	0.7	25.6	7.0	-3.8
1975—6	3.7	1.9	-6.4	8.3	4.9
1976—7	0.4	-0.3	-2.7	3.0	-1.4
1977—8	0.4	-3.4	-7.7	3.6	-2.3
1978—9	4.0	2.1	3.4	7.7	0.4
1979—80	2.1	1.2	3.8	3.1	4.5
1980—1	1.4	0.7	3.5	1.7	3.0
1981—2	2.0	0.6	1.6	1.5	0.4
1982—3	2.0	0.0	1.3	1.2	0.0

Source: Cmnd 7439 and Cmnd 6393 (converted to 1978 survey prices). Northern Ireland figures added to GB programmes.

Because the expected shortfall and the contingency reserve is not added to the individual programme figures, the expenditure in some of these programmes may be rather lower in 1978–9, 1979–80 and 1980–1, and a little higher in 1982–3. The rates of increase may be rather lower in the earlier years of this period and higher in the later years.

The programme shown add up to nearly four fifths of total public expenditure.

Table 5: NHS and GDP — Changes in Relative Costs and Prices (for Figure 7.3)

	Percentage change from previous year	
Year	NHS total expenditure compared with GDP factor cost	NHS final consumption compared with total consumption with total consumers' expenditure
	(1)	(2)
1967	+ 1.8	+ 2.1
1968	+ 1.1	- 0.1
1969	+ 3.0	+ 1.0
1970	+ 2.0	+ 4.2
1971	- 0.5	+ 2.0
1972	+ 0.4	+ 3.5
1973	+ 2.3	+ 0.2
1974	+ 8.8	+ 9.4
1975	- 1.3	+ 1.9
1976	+ 1.5	—
1977	- 0.8	- 3.5
1978	+ 0.3	+ 2.3

Source: Column 1 derived by comparing implied price index in National Income Blue Book, 1978, Tab.e 2.5 (updated by CSO) with index implied by our Table 1, Cols. 1 and 2, with rough adjustment for exclusion of transfers from column 2.

Column 2 derived similarly from Table 2.5 and Table 9.2, updated.

Notes to Figure 7.4: Data from OECD, *Studies in Resource Allocation*, no. 5 (1977), pp. 10 and 28, which shows figures for these and some other countries, for years in the early 1960s and mid-1970s. Both this volume and no. 6, on public expenditure (1978), contain valuable commentaries. The basis of the figures is not reliably uniform.

Printed and bound by CPI Group (UK) Ltd, Croydon, CR0 4YY

17/10/2024

01775689-0007